BRAIN BOOSTERS

FOODS & DRUGS THAT MAKE YOU SMARTER

ARE YOU EXPERIENCING BRAIN-DRAIN?

INSTRUCTIONS: For each of the following statements, check a "T" in the box if the statement is true or "F" if it is false. Count up the number of Ts to get your score.

T   F

☐ ☐ 1. My memory is not as good as it used to be.

☐ ☐ 2. It is harder to do calculations in my head than it used to be.

☐ ☐ 3. It is harder to concentrate than it used to be.

☐ ☐ 4. I often feel fuzzy headed.

☐ ☐ 5. I can't handle stress as well as I use to.

☐ ☐ 6. I get depressed more often than I use to.

☐ ☐ 7. I end the day feeling exhausted more often than I use to.

☐ ☐ 8. I often have a ringing sound in my ear(s).

☐ ☐ 9. I often drink so much coffee that I feel jittery and irritable.

☐ ☐ 10. It is harder to learn new things than it used to be.

☐ ☐ 11. I sometimes get lost while driving a familiar route.

☐ ☐ 12. I often tell the same stories over to the same people during short period of time.

☐ ☐ 13. I sometimes get confused over what time it is or where I am.

☐ ☐ 14. I often forget important appointments.

☐ ☐ 15. Lately I've had difficulty naming objects I'm familiar with.

IF YOUR SCORE IS:

12–15 Your brain is running on empty. Better see your doctor. You can refuel your brain with foods, vitamins, and drugs that make you smarter.

9–12 Brain drain is a danger. Check your diet today. You can reduce brain drain with vitamins and brain foods.

5–8 Your brain is functioning okay. By eating and drinking smarter your brain can function at optimal levels.

BRAIN BOOSTERS

FOODS & DRUGS THAT MAKE YOU SMARTER

BY BEVERLY A. POTTER, PH.D. & SEBASTIAN ORFALI

WRITTEN WITH GINI GRAHAM SCOTT, PH.D., J.D.

•

INTRODUCTION BY WARD DEAN, M.D.

•

PREFACE BY ROSS PELTON, R.PH., PH.D.

RONIN PUBLISHING, INC. • BOX 1035, BERKELEY, CA 94701

BRAIN BOOSTERS: *Foods & Drugs That Make You Smarter*
ISBN: 0-914171-65-8
Copyright © 1993 by Beverly Potter & Sebastian Orfali

Ronin Publishing, Inc.
Post Office Box 1035
Berkeley, California 94701

Project Editors:	Sebastian Orfali and Beverly Potter
Manuscript Editors:	Aiden Kelley, Dan Joy, Ginger Ashworth, Ward Dean
Index:	Nancy Freedom
Cover Design:	Brian Groppe
Page Composition:	Generic Type
Typographic Output:	Generic Type
Draft Manuscript:	The first draft was created with Gini Graham Scott

Printed in the United States of America by Delta Litho
First printing 1993

9 8 7 6 5 4 3 2 1

U.S. Library of Congress Cataloging in Publication Data
Beverly Potter
    Brain Boosters
    1. Reference.   2. Health.
    I. Title.

PERMISSION NOTICES

The authors have made every effort to trace the ownership of all copyright and quoted material presented. In the event of any question arising as to the use of a selection, we offer our apologies for any errors or omissions that may inadvertently have occurred, and will make necessary corrections in future editions of this book.

Acknowledgment and thanks are due the following authors, photographers, illustrators, agents, and publishers for permission to use their materials:

• COVER: Photo of glass head by Ben Fink.

Kirlian photo from *High Voltage Photography*, ©1975 by Henry Dakin.

• CHAPTER 1: Photograph of pouring Smart Drink by Marc Geller.

• CHAPTER 2: "Human Brain" reprinted from *Secrets of Life Extension*, by John Mann, And/Or Press. ©1980 John Mann. Permission to reprint granted by Ronin Publishing, Berkeley, CA. All rights reserved.

"Synaptic Junction of a Nerve Cell" and "Release of Neurotransmitter into synaptic cleft" from *Mind Foods and Smart Pills: A Sourcebook For The Vitamins, Herbs, & Drugs That Can Increase Intelligence, Improve Memory, & Prevent Brain Aging*, by Ross Pelton. ©1989 by Montrose P. Pelton. Used by permission of Doubleday, a division of Bantam Doubleday Dell Publishing Group, Inc.

"Structure of Nerve Cells" from *Mind Foods and Smart Pills: A Sourcebook For The Vitamins, Herbs, & Drugs That Can Increase Intelligence, Improve Memory, & Prevent Brain Aging*, by Ross Pelton. ©1989 by Montrose P. Pelton. Used by permission of Doubleday, a division of Bantam Doubleday Dell Publishing Group, Inc.

• CHAPTER 3: "When To See A Doctor About Memory Loss" from *Reversing Memory Loss*, by Vernon H. Mark with Jeffrey P. Mark. ©1992 by Vernon Mark and Jeffrey Paul Mark. Reprinted by permission of Houghton Mifflin Co. All rights reserved.

TABLE OF CONTENTS

BIBLIOGRAPHY

DIRECTORY OF LIFE EXTENSION DOCTORS 203

SUPPLIERS & SERVICES

INDEX 247

PREFACE

Ross Pelton, Ph.D., R.Ph.

Beverly Potter and Sebastian Orfali have made an important contribution to preserving one of our most important and threatened resources—our brains. Their book, *Brain Boosters*, provides a wealth of information on a broad range of topics related to substances that enhance intelligence. In a style that is both readable and understandable, they give complete explanations for a wide range of cognitive enhancers including vitamins, herbs, amino acids, other accessory nutrients, and pharmaceutical drugs.

Their clear discussion of brain physiology and function sets the stage for describing how cognitive enhancers work. The explanation of how and why the brain ages makes it possible to understand how the substances they have written about help to slow down and prevent brain aging and senility.

Brain Boosters also gives an interesting overview of the history and sociological impact of this new area of science. We now see smart drinks being served at smart bars, the rave-party scene, and multilevel marketing companies selling smart drugs and nutrients,

The FDA, the AMA, and other agencies are fighting to suppress the spread of the movement. However, it appears that a momentum has been generated by the public's interest and desire to have access to these new and useful brain boosters that will be very difficult for the government to stop. One of the major issues at stake is the question of freedom of choice in matters pertaining to our own health.

This book provides insight into FDA's perspective and gives specific information about how to legally order and obtain the substances that are reviewed. More and more people are becoming interested in health and want to actively enhance their health and wellness.

Brain Boosters leads readers on a fascinating journey through the new world of foods and drugs that make you smarter. The book also gives readers the information they need to make informed decisions about the benefits of taking cognitive-enhancing drugs and substances. I recommend *Brain Boosters* to anyone who is concerned about becoming smarter and staying that way—a group that includes everyone I know.

Dr. Ross Pelton is a pharmacist, nutritionist, and health educator in San Ysidro, California, specializing in nontoxic alternative cancer therapies. He is the author of Mind Foods and Smart Pills *and* Revolution in Cancer Therapy: The Complete Guide to Current Alternative Cancer Treatments. *Dr. Pelton's forthcoming book,* How to Prevent Breast Cancer, *focuses on ways women can minimize their risks and prevent breast cancer through diet, lifestyle, and healthy living. As a health consultant, Dr. Pelton conducts biological age testing for his clients and gives lectures and seminars on important health topics including anti-aging and life extension. His workshop, "Health for Corporate America: It Makes Dollars and Sense," for business executives, is very popular.*

INTRODUCTION

Ward Dean, M.D.

Brain Boosters is the latest contribution to the expanding body of literature that confirms the growing importance and awareness of cognitive enhancing substances.

A question I am often asked by journalists who cover the "smart-drug scene" is, "who uses *smart drugs*"? Although ABC's *Nightline* estimated in 1990 that there were over 100,000 smart-drug users in the United States, they did not state just who these users are. TV news and "tabloid-news" programs often give the impression that users of smart drugs and nutrients are primarily attendees of "smart bars" (where drinks are made from cognitive-enhancing amino acids and other nutrients) and participants in the "rave scene." However, this group is only the "tip of the iceberg," and is in reality, only a small minority (perhaps 10 percent) of those who use cognitive enhancing substances on a regular basis. The reason for this misconception is that this group of "ravers" and smart-bar attendees provides the most sensationalist visual images for television.

However, there are three other groups that also use smart substances—and these are the real "backbone" of the smart-drug movement. The first (and largest) group comprises those ranging in age from about 35–55—the "baby boomers" or "yuppies." These are generally well-educated, highly motivated, competitive people whose successful livelihoods depend on their brain power. Many are professionals like computer programmers, writers, physicians, attorneys, and scientists, who are either trying to further improve their cognitive abilities, or prevent the inevitable *aging associated memory impairment* (AAMI) to which we are all susceptible.

The second group is comprised of healthy seniors. These are people who want to stay healthy, and who also want to prevent or ameliorate the effects of AAMI, or even more severe dementing illnesses. Often, they have added various smart drugs and nutrients to their health-oriented lifestyles.

The third group is comprised of those who are already suffering from AAMI, Alzheimer's disease, Parkinson's disease, or some other form of dementing illness. Often, it is the patients themselves (in the early stages of the illness) who still retain the insight to be aware of their progressively more seriously impaired cognitive abilities. They may begin taking smart substances on their own, or request them from a concerned family member. These family members realize that there are alternatives to merely "living with the disability" or, in very severe cases, sending the patient off to a nursing home where further deterioration is almost inevitable.

I believe that progress in the development of cognitive-enhancing substances will rapidly accelerate in the next decade, for a number of reasons. First, because of our growing understanding of the biological basis of memory and the causes of AAMI and the dementias. Second, as a corollary to this increased knowledge, will be the development of even better drugs than we have now to enhance cognitive performance and delay and counteract the ravages of aging. Third, is the increased realization of pharmaceutical companies of the tremendous profits to be made in this field. Fourth, will be the appreciation by insurance companies and the government that preventive medicine and effective treatment in the area of cognitive performance will be much cheaper in the long run than "institutionalization" of those with dementing illnesses. Furthermore, companies will find that enhancing the cognitive abilities of their older, more experienced workers, will enable them to capitalize on these workers' vast stores of knowledge, as well as to restore their cognitive efficiency to that of their more youthful (and less experienced) coworkers.

Application of the information in *Brain Boosters* will enable anyone to get a "running start" on this burgeoning field.

Dr. Ward Dean is the director of the Center for Bio-Gerontology and has been engaged in gerontological research since 1977. He is the author of Biological Aging Measurement—Clinical Applications, Smart Drugs & Nutrients *(with John Morgenthaler),* The Neuroendocrine Theory of Aging and Degenerative Disease *(with Vladimir Dilman),* Smart Drugs II *(with John Morgenthaler and Stephen Fowlkes), and has published over 60 articles and reviews for professional journals.*

AUTHORS' FOREWORD

Smart drugs, pills, drinks, nutrients, mind foods, and brain boosters have become a big business. They are claimed to make the mind work better,increase the blood flow to the brain, increase the metabolism rate in the brain cells, replace certain brain chemicals that may be depleted by aging or disease, and maintain the longevity and efficiency of the brain cells. Millions of people are taking them, more and more every day.

Signs of this phenomenon are everywhere. Go to one of the increasingly popular "rave parties," which have a following in major U.S. cities among the twenties set, and you'll find smart-drink "bars" and smart-nutrient "cafés" alongside the traditional liquor and cappuccino bars. Go to a health-food store, and you'll find intelligence-boosting drinks and nutrient products prominently featured. Smart drinks and brain boosters are turning up at fitness clubs and holistic-health fairs. Doctors and scientists working with an aging population are using intelligence-enhancing drugs to turn back the signs of aging and the diseases of senility, such as Alzheimer's. Multilevel and network marketing companies market mind foods Amway-style to millions. An estimated 140 different brain-enhancing compounds are in various stages of development by pharmaceutical companies in the U.S. and in other countries. Add to that hundreds of foods, herbs, and nutrients in varying amounts and combinations acclaimed as sources of brain power. *Fortune* magazine predicts this activity could swell into an industry worth more than 40 million dollars by the mid-1990s.

The widespread interest in intelligence-enhancing drugs and nutrients was captured in the Steven King thriller *Lawnmower Man*, in which a scientist used an intellectually impaired man as a subject. When injected with a special mind formula, the man becomes superintelligent. Unfortunately, in the film, this foray into increasing human intelligence to godlike levels turns out badly, as the formerly gentle and sweet man runs amok, using his new-found intelligence to kill with superhuman powers and, he hopes, to take over the world, before he is destroyed by the scientist.

All ages of people are showing a growing desire to reap the benefits of improved mental functioning. Reasons for this increasing interest are many. Today's information overload means that people need to know more just to cope with the volumes of information. The growing aging population means that more and more people are facing the decline of mental agility that comes with age. For example, 20 percent of the population over eighty is subject to Alzheimer's. Not too surprisingly, people want to prevent or reverse that decline. Another reason is the increased competitiveness of the workplace in a competitive global market, which means there's more incentive to know more in order to get ahead. People want to up their brain power to do better in tests at school or on the job, for example. People often want to be smarter in order to be more interesting as conversationalists and to do better in social situations. Some people use brain boosters to repair the damage done to their brains by cigarette smoking, recreational drugs, pollutants, and normal aging. And now that smart drinks, drugs, and nutrients are becoming increasingly trendy, some people want to use them to be "in" and "with it."

WHAT CAUSES "BRAIN-DRAIN"?

As the brain ages, brain cells are less able to secrete chemicals, called neurotransmitters, needed to transmit electrical signals. The loss may come about because brain cells, called neurons, have died or because the spaces between the neurons, called synapses, have shrunk. Another cause is a lower level of neurotransmitters and other important chemicals in the brain, which inhibits the encoding of memories and slows recall.

NERVE-CELL DEATH

A process called oxidation destroys brain cells and creates free radicals as a by-product. Free radicals are killer molecules that kill cells, including neurons, and destroy neurotransmitters—which are the chemicals that transmit electrical messages from one brain cell to another. Researchers believe that free radicals cause many of the signs of aging, such as wrinkles and liver spots, chronic degenerative diseases, and decline in memory and mental functioning. Certain readily available vitamins, minerals, and nutrients are antioxidants that slow the oxidation process and reduce free radical damage.

Oxidation is caused by ordinary metabolic activities in the body, by eating animal fats and fats which are rancid or that have been overheated, by smoking, by inadequate oxygen, and by pollutants.

LOSS OF VITAL NEUROCHEMICALS

Brain cells need certain chemicals to transmit messages from one cell to another. These chemicals can be used up by unrelenting stress and destroyed by free radicals and oxidation. Many diets do not provide adequate amounts of the nutrients to produce the chemical neurotransmitters needed for optimal brain functioning.

OXYGEN STARVATION

Brain cells need adequate supplies of oxygen to function properly. When oxygen to the brain is reduced, free radicals are produced and brain cells die. Chronic lung disease and smoking deprives the brain of oxygen and kills brain cells.

CELLULAR GARBAGE BUILD UP

The waste product left over from cellular activity is called lipofusion. It remains as a deposit in the brain cells. It inhibits electrical activity in brain cells and can cause them to die.

• • •

Brain Boosters is a guide to the smart drugs and nutrient phenomena. The following chapters describe how the brain works and what causes mental decline. It tells what substances people are taking to increase their intelligence, explains how these substances act in the brain, and describes the most important brain-boosting drugs, vitamins, nutrients, and herbs. It chronicles the rising interest in brain boosters within both the underground "rave" culture and the performance-oriented mainstream. One chapter takes a look at the business side of the smart phenomenon; another recounts the controversy currently raging over the FDA's role in regulating vitamins. Finally, a directory provides a listing of doctors and clinics experienced in life extension, including cognitive-enhancement therapy.

Beverly A. Potter holds a Doctorate in counseling psychology from Stanford University and a Masters in vocational rehabilitation from San Francisco State University. Beverly provides consulting, training and public speaking for a wide range of organizations including Stanford University, Hewlett-Packard, GTE, SUN, TRW-CI, IRS, Becton Dickinson, and Genentech. Her books include Beating Job Burnout, Preventing Job Burnout, The Way of the Ronin, Turning Around, Drug Testing at Work, *and the forthcoming* Finding a Path with a Heart.

Sebastian Orfali holds a Masters in philosophy from University of New Mexico. Sebastian has twenty years experience in publishing. He has published over 100 books, primarily on health and psychoactive substances, including Holistic Health Handbook, Secrets of Life Extension, Psychedelics Encyclopedia, Your Body Works, New Healers, Controlled Sustances, Drug Testing at Work, Joyous Childbirth, *and* Smart Ways to Stay Young & Healthy.

I

FROM RAVE TO MAINSTREAM

Several trends intersect to create the smart phenomenon: the use of smart drugs, mind foods, and brain boosters. Gerontologists are using smart pharmaceuticals to counter aging and age-related diseases of mental decline. In a closely related development, middle-aged baby-boomers concerned with staying young and staving off the onset of aging are using brain boosters to increase their health and well-being. Another trend is the use of smart products to increase performance, from the classroom to the executive suites. Finally, the smart bars and nutrient cafés springing up in the "rave scene" appeal to an emerging new youth culture.

A person may consume smart foods for a variety of different reasons. Research on smart drugs got much of its initial impulse from gerontologists trying to sharpen the acuity of older people suffering from mental decline. But the applications of improving mental sharpness were quickly adopted by people concerned with health and performance, as well as those exploring the recreational possibilities of brain boosters. A rising executive, for example, may pop smart pills to be more alert and productive on the job, take smart nutrients to promote her health, and down a smart drink or two at a rave club in order to have the energy to dance until the wee hours of the morning.

People wonder if the benefits are real or just plain hype. The research is still coming in. However, scientists and medical practitioners have found evidence that smart nutrients and pharmaceuticals do have many of the health, performance, and anti-aging benefits claimed. At the same time, people using them for recreational purposes report experiencing more energy and having more fun.

HEALTH AND ANTI-AGING

It's hard to distinguish between the health and the anti-aging uses of the smart drugs and nutrients. People using supplements to be healthier also use them to stay younger and livelier and to stave off the mental and physical deterioration that come with age. The same people may use brain boosters to improve performance. On the other hand, professional researchers, scientists, medical practitioners, and gerontologists specializing in the treatment of the elderly are using the smart drugs and nutrients to combat symptoms of aging.

WHAT ARE SMART DRUGS?

Steven Fowkes, editor of *Smart Drug News*, defined smart drugs as any drug (or nutrient) that enhances aspects of mental performance. When we speak of "cognitive enhancement," we wish to include all of the myriad of mental functions that go into making us what we are. This would not only include such obvious aspects as intelligence and memory, but [also include] such items as sex, relaxation, sleep, immune function, and neuroendocrine regulation. These are all vital aspects of human health and well-being that are related to the functioning of the brain.

Steven Wm. Fowkes
Smart Drug News

The benefits of nutritional supplements traditionally have been confined to the fringes of acceptability. But recent research supports the claims that nutrients, especially vitamins, can protect against a host of ills ranging from birth defects and cataracts to heart disease and cancer.

Even more provocative to people over forty are glimmerings that vitamins can stave off the normal ravages of aging. Traditionally, pharmaceutical companies and medical practitioners have been wary of claims such as those of Linus Pauling about the benefits of vitamin C as a panacea for everything from colds to cancer. Further, pharmaceutical companies haven't done much research on vitamins, which are in the public domain, and can't be patented. Attitudes are shifting, however. There is growing acceptance of the efficacy of vitamins, nutrients, and smart drugs. In addition, growing use is creating a multibillion-dollar industry.

Another force driving the popularity of brain boosters is increased research attention. This has paved the way for greater acceptance. Medical focus in the 1980s changed from treating acute illnesses to caring for chronic diseases, such as heart disease and cancer, which are causing soaring health-care costs. In reaction, people sought less-expensive ways to treat and prevent chronic diseases. In this context, medical practitioners began recognizing that foods and vitamins can help people stay healthier longer, saving billions of dollars in health care and enabling people to live more satisfying lives.

Substantial research data since the 1970s support the relationship between diet and good health. Worldwide population studies consistently found that certain types of diets, most notably those with lots of fruits and vegetables, are associated with lower rates of chronic disease, such as cancer and heart disease.

Since the 1980s, there has been growing support for the theory that certain vitamins are *antioxidants*, which counteract destruction of cells and cell membranes by interfering with the action of naturally occurring toxic oxygen by-products called *free radicals*. Like molecular renegades, free radicals wreak havoc on cells by damaging DNA, altering biochemical compounds, corroding cell membranes, and destroying fats and proteins that are vital to the operation of cells. Free radicals are believed to underlie the gradual deterioration that is the hallmark of aging in all individuals, healthy as well as sick, and to play significant roles in age-related syndromes such as Alzheimer's and Parkinson's.

Research strongly suggests that antioxidants help stem the damage by neutralizing free radicals. Like cellular sheriffs, antioxidants collar the free radicals and haul them away. The discovery of antioxidants' effect was important to the development of the smart-drugs and nutrients movement. The battle against cell destruction occurs not only in the body as a whole, but in the brain as well, and so led to the conjecture that consuming antioxidants could improve brain power.

No wonder people get excited about the health and anti-aging possibilities of the brain boosters! The population is aging, and there are health risks caused by the deteriorating environment, including the degradation of the ozone, pollution caused by car exhausts, and the toxic wastes from manufacturing. Nutrient-supplement enthusiasts have touted nutrient supplements as an antidote for environmental and health problems as well as to stem the ordinary declines due to age.

PERFORMANCE

Desire to improve performance is an important reason for the growing interest in brain boosters. Stories abound of people who have achieved tremendous feats as a result of using brain boosters. *Intelli-Scope: The Newsletter of the Designer Foods Network* relates the story of the 55-year-old race driver, Mickey Thompson, who won the hazardous Baja 1000 off-the-road auto race. It was truly a test of endurance. For sixteen consecutive hours, he braved the hazards of a rough natural road course littered with large rocks that could easily damage his vehicle, as well as testing his nerves and his ability to concentrate. He had to make millions of quick decisions (about two or three per second) and could easily have suffered mental exhaustion from the intense concentration needed to do this. A momentary lapse in attention might have resulted in losing control of the vehicle.

Most race drivers ride with a co-driver, so that they can rest and restore their mental and physical energy. But Mickey successfully drove the entire race by himself. A key reason he was able to do so, the article relates, was his use of a high-energy drink developed by life-extension experts Durk Pearson and Sandy Shaw. Mickey kept a bottle taped to the steel crash cage of his car with a tube running from it to his mouth, so he could drink a little when he needed an extra energy charge.

Mickey is just one of many people who have turned to brain boosters to improve performance and health. Other examples include students who need to boost themselves up for a study session; a businessman who wants to put on a dynamite performance for a client; a speaker who must stimulate a large audience after a six-hour red-eye flight; a politician who has yet another whistlestop performance to make. Many people experimenting with brain boosters want to be better competitors. "It makes me feel more alert"; "I feel sharper"; "It helped me shake a hazy, fuzzy feeling" are the kinds of things people say about taking brain boosters.

Many fear falling behind in the competitive race if they don't do this. Mark Rennie, the co-founder of Smart Products, observed in an article

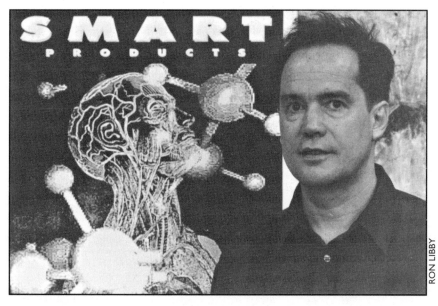

RON LIBBY

UPGRADING YOUR BRAIN: Mark Rennie, co-owner of Smart Products of San Francisco, was an early proponent of smart drinks and nootropics. He describes the boost he gets from smart drinks this way: "When I think of taking smart drugs, I feel like I'm upgrading a computer. Like going from a 286 chip to a 486."

in *Gentleman's Quarterly* that people who don't try to boost their productivity and energy are going to fall behind. "Everybody else is taking them . . . in Europe and Japan, they're going to be so far ahead of us in twenty years, that they'll just bury us. America will be worse than the third world."

Many people use smart nutrients in response to a speeded-up, overloaded modern age. We are all suffering from information and activity overload: so much to do; so little time to do it. The brain boosters may enable us to do more, concentrate better, speed up response time, and stay awake longer to accomplish more.

There are less personal reasons for the increasing desire to improve performance. Many people are responding to the competition that the U.S. is facing, where there is more and more pressure to do better. People are seeking that extra edge through any means possible, including consuming smart drugs and nutrients.

Smart drinks and brain boosters have been enthusiastically embraced by the younger generation. According to research scientist Sandy Shaw, author of the best-selling book *Life Extension*, people in their early twenties worry about economic survival and turn to brain boosters as a way to jump-start productivity and overcome the stress of competition. Sandy Shaw's co-author and fellow research scientist, Durk Pearson, says "these kids are under a hell of a lot of stress." This is the first generation in U.S. history that cannot count on achieving a higher standard of living than their parents. They feel under great pressure to get ahead and make it. There's a feeling that only the strongest and most resourceful will succeed. About this pressure, Pearson says, "In order to succeed during these highly competitive times, you need to increase your productivity, your stamina, your ability to work very long hours, and your ability to withstand stress. When nobody's taking care of you, and you've got to earn your own living in the middle of a recession or a depression, you've got to put your nose to the grindstone. And the faster you can turn that grindstone (or repair your nose), the farther you'll go."

The smart drugs and nutrients are a tool to achieve this end. After writing *Life Extension*, authors Pearson and Shaw developed a line of smart products to help increase individual productivity. Describing their nutrient combinations as "work-ethic formulations," Durk and Sandy said, "We specifically designed them to help us work longer, harder, more accurately, and more productively, and still have some energy left over afterwards for having fun." *Mondo 2000* editor, R. U. Sirius, called smart drugs "steroids for stockbrokers."

FLAWED CONCEPT

One of the flawed concepts is that drugs used to help correct dysfunctional brain conditions such as epilepsy or dementia can somehow elevate normal brain functioning to a smarter, "better-than-normal" state.

FDA Talk Paper

A growing body of research supports the effects of nutrients on mental performance. Dr. Dieter Bonke of the Merck Pharmaceutical Company in Germany, found in 1987 that the vitamins B_1, B_6, and B_{12} helped to increase the scores of marksmen shooting at targets. Over an eight-week period, the group taking the vitamins generally did better, and experienced less of a drop due to the stress of competition. *Smart Drugs and Nutrients* authors Dr. Ward Dean and John Morgenthaler say this study was "the first clear evidence under double-blind conditions of improved mental functioning of the central nervous system through the use of higher-than-recommended levels of vitamins." Subsequent research that confirmed that brain boosters can aid performance fueled interest. This sentiment was captured by Richard Guilliat who said in *Gentleman's Quarterly* that people are now looking for "better brains through chemistry. . . What humans need is a lean, mean, megabyte-crunching brain to cope with the daily motherlode of information."

THE RAVE SCENE

Recreational use of brain boosters to have more fun by being more alert, and to counter damage done by taking drugs and partying hard is popular among young people in the rave scene. The scene can be best described as a wild dance party. Raves are often held in a cavernous warehouse. Ravers dance all night to a throbbing mix of techno-pop called "house music." Psychedelic fractals and video images pulsate on the walls. People in all manner of costumes dance and gyrate to the beat pounding so strong you can't tell it from your own heart beat. *Newsweek* described the atmosphere as a "Freudian dream become real," in which people can play out their most far-out fantasies in the huge warehouses and dance clubs where these events take place.

Many of the ravers themselves, however, believe that the raves have a social significance far exceeding that of mere parties. As the *San Francisco Weekly* put it, "the people throwing these parties believe that they are a vanguard for a new society." One young raver was even quoted

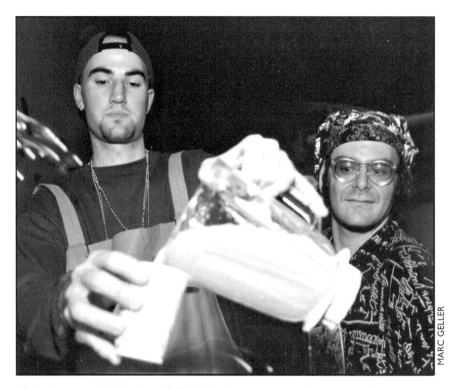

Chris Beaumont's Nutrient Café. Chris Beaumont watches bartender pour a smart drink at the Toon Town's New Year's Eve Rave in San Francisco.

saying, "In the next decade, there is going to be a total revolution of the mind." No doubt the mind revolution predicted by this raver was to draw its fuel from the brain boosters so prominent at the raves. A New Year's Eve party in San Francisco produced by the rave collective, Toon Town, was described by Cynthia Robbins in *Image Magazine*: "The lights synch with the sound—pulsing, whipping, whirling. Video screens televise live crowd shots overlaid with psychedelic fractal patterns. Laser-green light rays explode on the floor like shattered snakes. Smoke machines spew faux fog through which Intellebeam spots direct shards of color and white light, fragmenting on bodies, walls, and ceilings. . . The total sensory environment wraps the dancers in a techno-cocoon. It is disco inferno, psychedelic apocalypse. . . All around you are heaving bodies. . . The straight, the gay, the old, the young. Mostly young. A phantasmagoria hurled from the bar scene in *Star Wars.*"

Raves started in Europe in the late 1980s. By 1990 it was all the rage in England. About 15,000 or more partygoers might turn out on a given night dancing wildly, even in the open fields. The British Parliament cracked down, fearing the trend was getting out of hand. So the British ravers headed for San Francisco and Hollywood. They started the party circuit anew, passing out fliers in trendy stores letting people know where to find the "map point" for the next rave. The map point might be a Loony Toon ice-cream truck parked at the corner of Harrison and Third at 11 P.M. There, after paying an entrance fee, ravers receive a map to the party in a warehouse on the waterfront.

From Hollywood and San Francisco, the party scene spread to San Diego, New York, and other major cities around the country. Internationally, raves started popping up in such far-flung locations as Bangkok in Thailand, Tokyo in Japan, Goa in India, and the island of Ibiza in Spain. By 1992, the rave wave was coming aboveground. Commercial dance clubs and other promoters quickly capitalized on a popular trend. Entrepreneurial ravers like Toon Town lead the way, much as Bill Graham did in the 1960s when he commercialized the psychedelic hippie rock scene in the Fillmore and Avalon Ballroom. Raves have much the same feeling, although with the mixture of the high-tech synergized with '60s psychedelica.

Use of the drug MDMA or "Ecstasy" by ravers is common. Ravers worrying about the negative side effects of MDMA and wanting to have enough energy to dance until dawn often take smart drinks to decrease the nutrient and electrolyte depletion that may be caused by MDMA. Some of the smart drinks even contain large quantities of the amino acids used by the body in manufacturing the brain chemicals that some scientists believe are used up by the Ecstasy high. Smart drinks are claimed to improve concentration, short-term memory, and mental acuity; so the ravers believed they could enjoy what they are experiencing even more.

Smart bars became a standard feature at most raves. Ravers steeped themselves on smart drinks instead of imbibing "dumb" alcoholic drinks. With names like Psuper Psonic Psybertonic, Intellex, and Energy Elixir, smart drinks combine orange and other juices for flavoring, along with nutrients ranging from vitamins and minerals to phenylalanine, choline, and herbal extracts. Smart bars and nutrient cafés became profit centers. Toon Town, for example, served about 2,000 drinks and grossed more than $5,000 at the Nutrient Café run by Chris Beaumont on New Year's Eve of 1991.

The dance, the lights, the action, the sense of a unified community or "tribe" create a sense of oneness with hearts, minds, and bodies linked through the rhythmic throbbing energy of the music. Smart drinks became an important part of this phenomenon. It wasn't just that these concoctions helped the ravers keep up the energy to dance until the early morning hours. More importantly, they provided healthy alternatives to alcohol and the other "usual" drugs whose effects would have interfered with, rather than enhanced, the rave atmosphere of friendliness, openness, empathy, and positive community interaction.

In summary, a broad variety of needs and pressures from very different directions have combined to form a widespread interest in brain-boosting drugs and nutrients—and a rapidly expanding market for such products. These factors include issues of serious medical and social significance, such as the quest to cure age-related diseases and the need for a sharper "competitive edge" in a society under increasing economic pressure. But they also include purely personal goals such as the hope of enhancing health and extending life—or just extending one's endurance on the dance floor.

The smart phenomenon closes the distance between the corporate boardroom, the gerontology clinic, and the all-night dance club. A common ground has emerged between stressed-out executives, a new counterculture of freewheeling youths, and those afflicted by the ravages of aging: the desire for a better brain.

2

HOW THE BRAIN WORKS

Smart nutrients and brain boosters increase mental abilities by acting directly on the brain itself. Understanding how the brain works provides a clearer picture of how these substances affect the brain to improve mental functioning.

HOW THE BRAIN FUNCTIONS

According to scientists, the brain consists of about 100 billion individual nerve cells called *neurons*. This estimate has risen steadily over the years, and is ten times higher than it was two decades ago, when there were thought to be around only 10 billion cells in the brain. It staggers the imagination to think of the possibility that, as time goes by, the figure may well continue to go up!

Neurons are clumped together like masses of trees in a tropical rain forest. Extending from them are long, thick branches that reach out like vines called *axons*. Axons transmit electrical signals from one neuron to another, much as a telephone switching system sends a call from one place to another.

Like most cells, neurons are electrically charged. There is a very small difference, of about 75 millivolts, in the amount of electrical energy from one side of the cell membrane to the other. Negatively charged molecules are concentrated inside the cell, and more positively charged atoms outside.

What is unique about the neurons, in contrast to other kinds of cells, is that they can detect very small electrical currents and transmit them to other cells. As Dr. Ross Pelton, author of *Mind Foods and Smart Pills*, who conducts biological age testing for his clients notes, "It is the flow of these bioelectrical currents that determines the thought processes of the brain."

MASTER CONTROL CENTER

The brain is the master control center of your whole body. It consumes 25 percent of all metabolic energy, and the six billion nerve cells it contains make up half the body's total nerve cells. It stimulates motor functions, digestion, growth, and tissue repair; it interprets your sensory experiences and decides which physical and emotional responses to make.

Yet, despite this incredible power, your brain constitutes only 2 percent of your body's weight. This makes it highly sensitive: nutritional deficiencies can cause brain imbalances that send shock waves through your entire body, resulting in everything from fatigue and forgetfulness to depression and anxiety.

Robert Erdmann
The Amino Revolution

The neuron normally exists in a resting state, called *resting potential*, in which a biological pump in the cell wall maintains a slight negative charge inside by pushing the positively charged atoms out of the cell. When the neuron is stimulated along the tree-like projections from the neuron, called *dendrites*, it becomes electrically excited. Then the electrical charge within the cell increases, so that the inner electrical charge becomes positive, rising to about +50 millivolts. The active charge, called the *action potential*, spreads along the cell wall into the long axon, which reaches out to other cells. In this way, the action potential enables one neuron to convey its message through

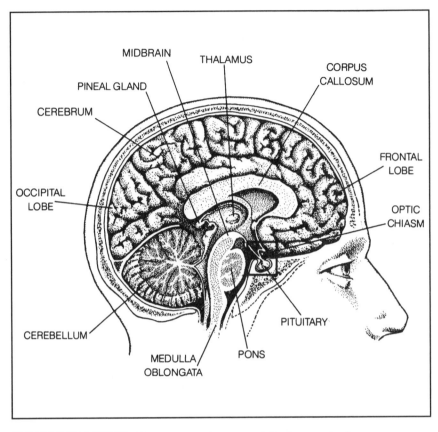

THE HUMAN BRAIN: Master control center of the human body.

electrical signals to others, which in turn transmit that message on to still other neurons throughout the brain.

The process works a little like a relay switching station at the phone company. When a signal comes in for a call, it triggers switches in one location, which trigger switches in another switching center, and the call goes though, all in a matter of seconds. The neurons in the brain do their switching and signaling thousands of times faster, and there are many more signals pouring through simultaneously when we're thinking.

THE STRUCTURE OF NEURONS

Because neurons are central to the system, it helps to understand how the neuron is structured and what the different parts do to make the process work. Like other cells, the neuron has the usual cell body and nucleus. But in addition, reaching out from the cell body, are long tree-like structures called *dendrites* that receives and sends signals through a *synaptic end bulb* on the axon. The juncture where the end bulb of one axon transmits a signal to the dendrites of another nerve cell is called the synaptic junction, or *synapse*.

The signal itself is a simple on-off charge, like a yes or no in a computer. Operating like a relay switching system, the signal travels

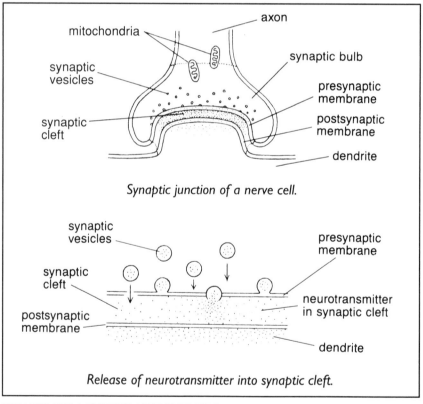

Synaptic junction of a nerve cell.

Release of neurotransmitter into synaptic cleft.

FROM *MIND FOOD & SMART PILLS: A SOURCEBOOK FOR THE VITAMINS, HERBS, & DRUGS THAN CAN INCREASE INTELLIGENCE, IMPROVE MEMORY, & PREVENT BRAIN AGING* BY ROSS PELTON. COPYRIGHT ©1989 BY MONTROSE P. PELTON. USED BY PERMISSION OF DOUBLEDAY, A DIVISION OF BANTAM DOUBLEDAY DELL PUBLISHING GROUP, INC.

from one axon through a synapse to a dendrite on another neuron. Sometimes these axons between neurons can be very long, about three feet or more, and the signal can travel at varying speeds, measured in milliseconds. The axons vary, too, depending upon whether they are insulated or not, which affects speed. Generally the shorter axons or axons from nerve centers, such as the stomach, are uninsulated, so that the speed of transmission is a little slower. But in longer axons, or axons from centers where the speed of information is more critical, such as the hands or feet, which we must move quickly, the axon is normally insulated by a covering of specialized cells made up of myelin. The *myelin sheath*, which is a little like the insulation of an electrical wire in a house, helps to speed the transmission along the nerve.

Just imagine: the brain has billions of cells with their dendrites, axons, and synaptic end bulbs all packed together and interconnected with one another, reaching out beyond the brain with the vine-like axons to nerve cells throughout the body. Trillions of interconnections are possible as the various nerve cells alternate between being at rest and firing off electrical messages, which turn neighboring nerve cells on or off.

MAKING CONNECTIONS: LIFE IN THE FAST SYNAPSE LANE

While the neuron sends out and receives messages, synapses, which are the spaces between the receiving dendrites and sending axons, are critical to how quickly and clearly messages are received. It is like putting a plug in an electric socket. There has to be a good connection for the electricity to flow through. If anything interferes with the connection, lights can dim or go off. If the circuit gets overloaded, a circuit could be shorted out.

A close-up look at synapses shows a small end bulb, or *synaptic terminal*, in which there are small, round containers called *synaptic vesicles* that contain special *neurotransmitter chemicals* that facilitate the electrical flow of messages across the synapse. Depending on the chemical composition of the neurotransmitters, electrical flow will be

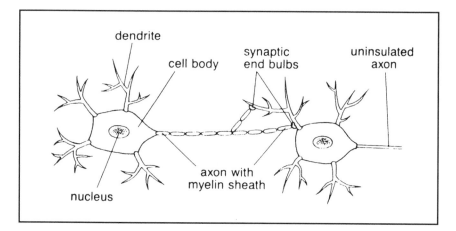

SYNAPTIC JUNCTION: Structure of nerve cells.

faster or slower. Brain boosters can be used to improve the chemical mix of neurotransmitters to speed up the flow of information.

Here's what happens as a message crosses the synapse. When an electrical current arrives at a synapse, the synaptic vesicles move toward the membrane of the synaptic end bulb at the end of the axon and release their neurotransmitter chemicals, which then flow through the *presynaptic membrane* of the end bulb into the *synaptic junction*, which is the space between the axons of one neuron and the dendrites of another.

On the other side of the synaptic junction, the neurotransmitting chemicals come to the membrane on the dendrite called the *postsynaptic membrane* that picks up the incoming message, to be passed on in the same way from the axons of that nerve cell across another synaptic junction to the dendrites of another neuron.

The place where a neurotransmitter released by the axon of one neuron binds to the dendritic membrane of another neuron is called a *receptor site*. The neurotransmitter fits into the receptor site like a key fitting into a lock. Just as a lock will accept only a certain key, receptor sites are shaped so that only specific neurotransmitters will be able to bind to them.

Another way to look at neurotransmission is to imagine that the synapse is a river running between two shores or brain cells. The end bulb on the axon is like the dock from which the boat departs. The receptor site is the dock on the other side of the river, where the boat unloads its message.

HOW THE BRAIN GROWS AND CHANGES

The neurons in the brain are called *postmitotic cells*, because they don't multiply after the brain structure is originally created. According to aging researcher Albert Rosenfeld, once such cells die, they are "dead and gone forever." (As we will see later, however, there is some recent evidence that, under the right conditions, the brain can, in fact, grow new cells.) In other words, over time, the brain gradually loses nerve cells with their synaptic connections, because of normal wear and tear, accidental injury, aging, or strokes. The actual extent and effect of brain cell loss are in dispute. Researchers once believed that in the normal course of aging as many as 100,000 brain cells were lost every day after age 35. Although it is generally believed that there is brain-cell loss over time, this high figure has been challenged by Alex Comfort, one of the world's leading gerontologists. Enthusiasts for smart drugs and nutrients assert that aging due to nerve-cell loss can be slowed by the use of brain boosters, nutrients, and drugs.

A second site of decline is the dendrites, which receive messages from other cells. Dendrites are very fragile and easily damaged. Thus, apart from specific injuries or disease, simple biological aging can reduce the number of dendrites, leading to reduced connections and communications between brain cells, resulting in a corresponding decline in intelligence that can progress to senility with aging. Researchers believe that by protecting the dendrites from damage, intelligence can be preserved.

New research indicates that brain cells or neurons may change in response to experience. Brain-booster enthusiasts believe that smart drinks, drugs, and nutrients can be used to facilitate this change.

Researchers have found that the dendrites can grow new protrusions in minutes in response to new experiences. New impressions, such as sights, sounds, thoughts, smells, can contribute to the creation of new synapses as the electrical signals generated by these experiences cause the release of neurotransmitter chemicals. When the memory of a particular experience is recorded, the electric pulses representing the event leads to the creation of new synapses dotted with the synaptic vesicles that release neurotransmitters. Thus, as you learn and have new experiences, the very structure of your brain actually changes. To return to the analogy of the phone relay station, when the brain grows new connections, it's as if more wires have been added to the phone system to allow you to call up new numbers and so to access new information.

THE CONGESTED BRAIN THEORY

In the 1970s, William Bondareff and Robert Narotzky of the Northwestern University Medical School in Chicago looked inside the brains of rats, at the spaces between the cells. When they measured those spaces, they found that they were only about half as wide in older rats as they were in their younger counterparts. It may be that these spaces are akin to Los Angeles freeways, in that they are the "roads" along which travel the vital chemicals that are the brain's messengers. As anyone who lives in Los Angeles knows, when you narrow the freeway, even by one lane, you get horrible traffic jams, and everybody's late to work. It could be that just this sort of thing is going on in the aging brain. And if the messengers—the neurochemicals— get bogged down because of congestion, so does the brain. Since much of the rest of the body needs the brain to tell it what to do, when the brain gets jammed, the body has a rough time processing its workload.

Kathy Keeton
Longevity: The Science of Staying Young

The number of connections made by a single neuron are phenomenal. According to brain researchers, a single neuron can have as many as 100,000 synapses connecting it with its neighboring neurons. There may be as many as 100 billion neurons in the brain—researchers aren't exactly sure how many, though this is a common estimate—the number of connections, reflecting the number of neurons multiplied by the number of synapses, is in the trillions. As a result, the individual can make intuitive connections not yet possible in computers. These many connections mean that there is a redundancy of information spread around the brain. If one part of a brain is damaged, the information or memory will be contained and can be accessed elsewhere. It is believed that consuming smart drinks and drugs increases the number of connections, resulting in increased capacity.

CHEMICALS IN THE BRAIN

Neurotransmitters are responsible for the transmission of electrical signals in the brain from neuron to neuron. Other chemicals in the brain, called *neurohormones*, promote its functioning. Researchers believe that certain nutrients, primarily amino acids, form the precursors or building blocks that the body uses to manufacture brain chemicals. This process also requires the participation of other nutrients. The precursor nutrient is like the clay used to make a sculpture. But the artist and his tools—a team of other nutrients—are still required in order for the final sculpture, or molecule, to take shape. Thus it makes sense that we should be able to increase our brain power by consuming the right nutrients in the right combinations to make the right chemicals.

Acetylcholine. Acetylcholine is a neurotransmitter that is believed to play a crucial role in memory. It is produced by a complex chemical process in the end bulb of the axon from a combination of acetate and choline molecules. Imagine a small chemical factory within each nerve cell, shaped like a tiny egg, with a filament-like substance inside called the mitochondria. Glucose, for energy, and oxygen, which metabolizes the glucose, are taken from the blood and combined with acetate in a chemical process (the citric-acid cycle) to produce the enzyme acetyl coenzyme (or acetyl CoA) and adenosine triphosphate (ATP), a substance that provides energy in cells. Acetyl coenzyme combines with the choline molecules to create acetylcholine. Once created, this acetylcholine travels from the axon to the receptors in the dendrites, and triggers the electrical discharge. After being used, the acetylcholine is broken down again into acetate and choline by an enzyme called acetylcholinesterase or AChE. Once again, the acetate and choline are reabsorbed back into the end bulb to be recreated into acetylcholine through another cycle with more oxygen and glucose for energy. Besides their important role in the creation of acetylcholine, oxygen and glucose are energy sources and building blocks. It is believed that anything that increases the supply of oxygen and glucose or other chemicals in this mix contributes to making more acetylcholine, which facilitates transmission of electric current and boosts intellectual response.

Gamma-Aminobutyric Acid (GABA). This neurotransmitter acts like acetylcholine and other neurotransmitters; it crosses from the axon to the dendrite through the synaptic cleft in response to an electrical signal in the neuron. But unlike acetylcholine, which helps to transmit signals, GABA inhibits message transmission. This is important, because blocking transmission helps to control the nerve cells from firing too fast, which would overload and exhaust the system. Otherwise, according to Pelton, the neural networks would increasingly stimulate themselves and send signals faster and faster from one neuron to another until the whole system collapsed from exhaustion. So GABA helps to balance out the more rambunctious acetylcholine, a little like a shut-off valve on a heater that turns off when it becomes too hot.

Serotonin. This is another inhibitory neurotransmitter that contributes to slowing down the system. However, in contrast to acetylcholine and GABA, which are involved in transmitting or putting the breaks on the transmission of specific information, serotonin is a neurohormone that acts on the overall operations of the brain.

A chemical called tryptophan, found in foods such as bananas, turkey, and potatoes, is converted through a series of complex chemical processes into serotonin. Researchers have obtained some evidence that an increase in serotonin can produce sleep; thus foods high in tryptophan are likely to make you sleepy. It is also believed that this neurotransmitter may be "used up" or depleted by physiological processes that occur during sleep.

Serotonin is related to the brain's general state of alertness. It also plays an important role in pain regulation. Its most important job may be the part it plays in regulating mood. For example, low levels of serotonin have been linked to depression. The popular antidepressant drug Prozac works by preventing the reabsorption or "reuptake" of serotonin into brain cells, thus increasing the amount of serotonin active in the synapses.

Judging from this description, you may not think serotonin particularly useful for improving thinking. But one needs to be rested and in a good mood to think well, and serotonin contributes to this needed balance.

Dopamine. Dopamine is a chemical that acts like a neurohormone in contributing to the overall functioning of the brain. Specifically, it facilitates control of physical movement. Without dopamine, the body develops Parkinson's disease, which is characterized by tremors and repetitive movements. Dopamine is produced through a chemical reaction with its precursor, L-dopa. Researchers have found that L-dopa reduces or eliminates the tremors or repetitive-movement symptoms of Parkinson's disease. This was dramatically chronicled in the film *Awakenings,* in which actor Robin Williams played Dr. Oliver Sachs, who got dramatic results by treating chronic patients with L-dopa. Thus, brain-booster enthusiasts argue if someone has movement problems that interfere with functioning and straight thinking, an increase in supplements that produce dopamine in the body will help.

There are other interesting facts about dopamine. Excessive concentrations of dopamine in certain parts of the brain have been linked to mental disorders such as schizophrenia. It is believed that caffeine derives its stimulating effect from interacting with the brain's dopamine system. Since dopamine is related to movement, extremely high doses of caffeine can result in convulsions.

Norepinephrine. This neurohormone acts like a kind of amphet-amine or speed injection on the brain. Norepinephrine is produced in a small group of cells in the brain stem that release this hormone to the rest of the brain. Then, once released, like adrenaline, it stimulates the capillaries to expand so that more blood can flow through, which increases the blood to the brain. Pelton says it acts like an amphetamine on the nerve cells, which steps up brain activity and alertness. The norepinephrine molecule even bears a structural resemblance to am-phetamine molecules.

Norepinephrine appears in particularly high concentrations in the lower brain and brain stem. In his book *A Primer of Drug Action,* Robert M. Julien, M.D. states that because these parts of the brain "appear to be essential to the display of basic instinctual behavior in hunger, thirst, emotion, and sex, norepinephrine may be a neurotransmitter important in the regulation of those functions."

Since norepinephrine is considered an "excitatory" neurotransmit-ter, it is not hard to understand why levels of this brain chemical have been linked to the mental disorder of mania, which is characterized by a state of extreme overstimulation.

Endorphins. Endorphins are neurohormones described by re-searchers as a source of pleasure and reward, as well as a means of reducing one's awareness of pain and irritation. The body releases endorphins when it experiences stress or when one achieves a desired goal as a result of an action. They are feel-good chemicals that encourage motivation to continue doing or thinking about something. This stimulated interest and attention might, in turn, facilitate mental processing. After all, if one is focused and excited about something, one is bound to put in a better performance.

Endorphin molecules are similar in structure to opiate drugs such as morphine whose pain-killing and "feel-good" effects are believed to result from interaction with the brain's endorphin systems. We owe much of our understanding of neurotransmission and brain function, as well as drug action, to endorphins and a neuroscientist named Candace Pert. In the early '70s, Pert experimented with opiates and the endorphin system to confirm the existence of receptor sites in the brain, paving the way for many important subsequent discoveries.

CELLULAR GARBAGE THEORY

During the middle and late 1950s, a number of researchers noted that many cells, especially the nonreplicating cells of the brain and muscles, tend as they age to build up piles of chemical garbage, in particular, a pigmented fat called *lipofuscin*. In some of those cells the lipofuscin piles got so big that they took up as much as 30 percent of the cell's room.

Anyone who's ever been in New York City during a garbage strike can instantly see the power of both the analogy and the theory: garbage can indeed be paralyzing. On the level of the cell, it can cause cross-linking and other kinds of malfunctions that are among the signposts of aging.

Why is cross-linking so damaging? Think of a childhood game, the three-legged race. Two people running side by side, each using both legs freely, can run a competent fifty-yard dash. Take those same two people and tie one of their legs together, and not only are they substantially slowed, but they become so still that they may not be able to run at all. According to Bjorksten's theory, much the same thing happens when molecules inside the cells become cross-linked; the molecules, be they proteins or what have you, stiffen to the point that they eventually lose their ability to do their jobs. The result? Our now-familiar enemies, aging and death.

Kathy Keeton
Longevity: The Science of Staying Young

Lipofuscin. Lipofuscin is a left-over chemical from processes in cells as they react to the neurotransmitters and metabolize other chemicals. It is "cellular garbage," the waste product that is left over from cellular activity, and remains as a deposit in the brain cells. As deposits build up, they can inhibit and disrupt the normal processing or electrical activity in cells, including their ability to receive and transmit information. If the deposits increase enough, they can cause cells to die. Here again, smart drugs and nutrients can come to the rescue, by removing lipofuscin deposits and enabling cells to function effectively again.

BETTER THINKING THROUGH CHEMISTRY

Altering the chemical composition or balance within the brain can improve mental functioning. The trick is to find the chemicals or nutrients that influence the production of the neurotransmitters and neurohormones in the brain.

SENILE DEMENTIA

Although there are permanent losses of neuronal cells throughout life, these do not necessarily lead to mental incompetence. Even when large masses of brain tissue are destroyed or removed, the remaining cells can take over their functions, and the loss may be scarcely noticed. Nevertheless, there is often a reduction of mental capacity and intellectual energy in the aged. Rather than being the result of decreased numbers of brain cells, senile dementia appears to be due to changes in and around these cells.

John Mann
Secrets of Life Extension

An increase in chemicals or nutrients can have several kinds of effects. Some will not make much difference as long as one has enough for basic functioning. For example, eating more protein will not make you smarter, once your brain is operating at its usual level of functioning. In other cases, you may be able to overcome a deficiency that is interfering with ability to think properly. For example, if you don't have enough protein, your thinking processes may slow down or become confused, so that you can't think clearly or have the energy to think well. But if you eat more, you can reverse this process and think the way you normally do again. Sometimes thinking and other mental abilities can be improved by increasing the amount of some particular chemicals, such as choline, which is converted into the neurotransmitter acetylcholine.

NUTRIENTS & NEUROTRANSMITTERS

By maximizing the health and functioning of the neuron, we maximize the basic building block of mental performance and intelligence. Nutrients have a strong influence in this process of optimizing mental functioning. . . . Neurotransmitters are the "chemical messengers" that brain cells use to communicate with each other. . . . Several of the "smart pills" . . . work by increasing the level of these neurotransmitters."

Ross Pelton
Mind Foods and Smart Pills

Researchers have tested the effects of various chemicals on the brain by giving people different kinds of drugs or nutrients or by experimenting with animals and drawing inferences from changes in their behavior as to how individuals would be likely to be affected. For instance, if they find that a rat learns a maze better or a human can better memorize a list of words after being given a particular smart drug or nutrient, this suggests that the substance has somehow helped increase that animal or human's brain power.

The theory is that the substance had this effect because it improved chemical and/or electrical processing in the brain. In turn, because so many different chemical reactions and substances are involved in the process, smart drugs or nutrients can affect different processes differently, and any one or a combination of these things can contribute to the improvement. For example, some substances might improve mental functioning by improving the flow of oxygen to the brain; some might do so by improving the formation of memories, which are themselves created by electrical or chemical activity; and some might improve the flow of information to the brain by stimulating the transmission process, which is done by the neurotransmitters.

By understanding how the brain works, we can begin to understand how brain-boosting drugs and foods can improve our mental functioning. Most important to remember are the many significant roles played by brain chemicals such as acetylcholine, norepinephrine, and the others we have discussed in this chapter. Drugs can affect the levels of different chemicals in our brains; some drugs may even be able to mimic the actions of certain brain chemicals. And since the body manufactures brain chemicals from nutrients, ingesting various nutrients can also affect how well our brains work.

3

MEMORIES AND THOUGHTS

Knowing how the brain remembers and processes thoughts can help you to understand how brain foods and smart drugs contribute to better cognitive functioning. The previous chapter, on how the brain works, described nerve-cell structure, chemistry, and how brain boosters affect them. In this chapter, the focus is on how the brain processes memories and thoughts, and on how aging interferes with remembering and thinking.

Smart drugs and brain foods can affect the brain in a number of ways. It is a little like someone trying to improve the operations in an office. The structure can be changed. What's in the office and how it's arranged can be improved. Better equipment can be installed; desks can be moved around; and more skilled people can be hired. Alternatively, the process can be changed. The way the people work together can be improved to make them more efficient and productive. By using various smart drugs or nutrients, for example, people can improve memory and, therefore, how they think.

TYPES OF MEMORIES

We have four types of memory, and each of these can be affected by certain brain foods and smart drugs. Most people know about short-term and long-term memory. In the 1950s, a third type of memory, the working memory, was identified.

Short-term memory is in operation when you remember something for a matter of seconds, such as a name of a person you just met at a party or when you repeat back a telephone number. Then, after you leave the conversation at the party or finish making the phone call, you promptly forget that name or number. The impression has been entered into only your short-term memory, and it hasn't created a more permanent trace.

Long-term memory, by contrast, is that deeper impression that occurs when we experience or think about something enough that it, in effect, becomes etched into the operations of the nervous system, so that we can recall it at will.

MEMORY LOSS AND AGING

It is said that, in old age, the memory is the first mental capacity to go. Actually, it is the first loss that we notice. It is difficult to be aware of being more or less creative for most people. We do not notice the gradual loss of the sense of smell or a decrease in reasoning power. But we do notice when we are unable to recall recent events or the name of someone we met last week.

Ross Pelton
Mind Foods and Smart Pills

A good example of the difference between short- and long-term memory is the way a personal computer works. A short-term memory is like the preliminary impression made when you are first writing in a file. The impression is there long enough that you can print it out by pushing the print key, a little like focusing on that first impression, thought, or statement of a name or number that you hear and then repeat. But if you don't create a permanent file name and save what you have just written onto the disc, that unsaved file, like a preliminary impression, is lost for memory retrieval. It might be retrieved somehow by a special program designed to restore unsaved files, much as some special mental processing might be able to pull out a normally passing thought or short-term

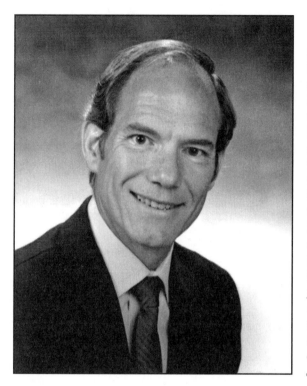

Ross Pelton, R.Ph., Ph.D., is a pharmacist, a nutritionist, and a health educator. He is the author of Mind Foods and Smart Pills and Revolution in Cancer Therapy: The Complete Guide to Current Alternative Cancer Treatments. Dr. Pelton is assistant administrator of the Hospital Santa Monica in Baja, Mexico. He gives seminars on anti-aging and life-extension and conducts biological age testing for his clients.

memory. But generally, such short-term memories quickly disappear, and perhaps for good reason. They aren't important enough to retain, and if we kept them all, we would overload our mental processes with too much data; similarly, if we tried to save everything on disc, we would soon overload the memory capacity. Or, as Pelton explains the process in *Mind Foods and Smart Pills*, the "short-term memories pass into some sort of temporary holding pattern in the brain, and those memories that are important to us are then passed on to permanent storage."

Working memory falls somewhere in between short-term and long-term memory. According to Pelton, it enables us to "store important information for a short period of time, recall it, and then forget it, if necessary." Working memory is called into operation when you meet someone at a party, have a brief conversation, and put that person out of mind. Later, someone asks you whom you met, and you suddenly recall that person's name. But the following day, any recall of that name is gone from memory, because remembering that person's name isn't important to you any more.

Vital memory is the core of memory and, according to Dr. Vernon Marks, author of *Reversing Memory Loss*, "it is at the core of your being, representing the essential you, your personality, your feelings." Vital memory is essential to functioning successfully in the world. Vital memory includes the memories laid down very early in life, such as when and how to use a toilet, how to dress and act in public, and rules of safety. When vital memory is damaged by a stroke or an accident, the person can have difficulty functioning independently.

HOW MEMORIES ARE FORMED AND RECALLED

Scientists are still debating exactly how memories are created and recorded in the brain. The most widely accepted theory is called the *synaptic alteration theory*. It postulates that a new stimulus triggers a change in the synapses of a neuron or a group of neurons. A short-term memory is recorded when the change is just a temporary or less-significant change, whereas a long-term memory results from a permanent and/or deeper change. The working memory is a transitional process that can revive a short-term temporary impression before it disappears, and can enter into the imprint of a long-term memory.

The neurotransmitter chemicals released in the synapses play a key role in the creation of memories. There is an interaction between the electrical signals in the brain and the amount of neurotransmitters released. Pelton points out that different electrical signals "lead to changes in the amount of neurotransmitter released and even a change in the effect of the released transmitter substance on the receptor site."

In turn, neurotransmitters have an effect on the passage of electrical signals through the neurons. A sufficient supply of needed neurotransmitters helps the neurons function effectively. In their best-seller *Life Extension*, researchers Durk Pearson and Sandy Shaw suggest that increased neurotransmitters can improve memory functioning. As they point out, neurotransmitters play a critical role in the memory creation and retrieval process, as well as in thinking, learning, and other bodily activities, because all these activities depend on the ability of the neurons in the brain to make and transmit neurotransmitters to other neurons.

As the brain ages, neurons are less able to secrete neurotransmitter chemicals and transmission of electrical signals is impaired as a result. The loss may come about because the brain loses neurons and the spaces between neurons declines. Another factor is a lower level of neurotransmitters and other important chemicals in the brain that leads to slow entry and processing of memories.

THE MYTH OF AGING

To understand aging we must understand the difference between chronological aging and biological aging. Chronological aging is simply the measurement of the passage of time. We will continue to have birthdays; the pages of the calendar will continue to turn.

Biological aging, however, is the gradual destruction of the human body. Most people believe that biological and chronological aging happen together. This is a myth. As we grow older with time, we do not have to destroy our bodies. In fact, we now know that biological aging can be slowed down; it can be stopped, and in some cases, it can even be reversed.

Ross Pelton
Mind Foods and Smart Pills

THE DECLINE IN NEURONS

A decline in the number of neurons affects memory because there are fewer neurons on which to impress memories, as well as fewer connections for retrieving these memories. The exact number of neurons lost is the focus of much debate. Researchers agree there is some neuron loss as we age, but they dispute the early estimates that the average woman or man permanently loses about 100,000 neurons a day after age 35. Some experts say that neuron loss is part of our normal programming, and point to normal wear and tear as the cause. Others blame neuron loss on a decline in efficient blood circulation, which results in less oxygen to the brain. Richard Dawkins, zoologist from Oxford, maintained that neurons are selectively chipped away through cell death as part of the formation of the personality and its memories, much as a sculptor chips away the unneeded bits of rock to create a sculpture.

However, whatever the reasons, researchers generally believe that the brain does lose some cells, though at varying rates in different parts of the brain, ranging from no loss in some areas to high levels of loss in others, so that over time, with aging, the brain functions less effectively. Brain weight drops about 10 percent overall by the age of eighty, according to the findings of Neal R. Cutler of the National Institute on Aging. He found the number of neurons declined as much as 25 percent in some areas, and the decline was associated with less neurochemical activity in these areas.

The brain functions less effectively in recalling memories as it loses cells, because the image, picture, or story making up that memory becomes less clear. What happens is that the impression of a particular memory is entered into a number of cells in various places around the brain and is then stored in these different areas. Moreover, many new memories can be formed simultaneously in different cells or groups of cells. Thus, there is no particular cell or specific circuit for any particular memory. In other words, the creation of memories seems to operate like the creation of a hologram, in which the memory is recorded in a number of places, so that it can be viewed or retrieved from a number of angles. In turn, the more entries for that memory, the clearer and stronger the image, and the easier it is to retrieve it. When cells or connections of cells are lost through the process of aging, one can still call up memories. People still remember particular memories when a part of the brain is cut out, for example. However, the memories become less clear and fuzzier when one tries to recall them.

One way to think of the process is to imagine a photograph that is reproduced through a screen. The more dots on the screen, the higher the resolution. Conversely, as there are fewer dots, the image becomes less clear. The creation and recall of memories in the brain seems to operate much the same way. The stronger the original image, the more neurons in the brain that contain it, and the stronger the memory. As the number of neurons impressed with that memory declines, so does the power of that memory.

DECLINE IN THE SIZE OF THE SPACES BETWEEN NEURONS

The size of the spaces between neurons also shrinks with aging. This shrinkage could account for the decline in the size of the brain with age. Harry Demopoulus, a pathologist at New York University, discovered from doing autopsies that the brains of very old people physically shrunk by as much as a third. Other researchers found this shrinkage in rat brains. William Bondareff and Robert Narotzky from the Northwestern University Medical School in Chicago measured the spaces between rat-brain cells and discovered that the spaces between cells in the brains of older, senescent rats were, on the average, only half as large as those in the brains of younger rats.

Researchers believe that this shrinkage has a negative effect on overall brain functioning, because the reduction of space increases pressure and density, which leads the neurons to perform normal cell activities less effectively. The intercell spaces are critical in transporting chemicals across the synapses, from neuron to neuron, which is essential to communication among neurons. Through this complicated communication process, the brain regulates all body functioning. Some researchers argue that the cell-space reduction is the root cause of aging throughout the body.

REVERSING LOSSES IN NEURONS, SPACES, AND CONNECTIONS

Brain foods slow the losses in neurons and the spaces between them by replenishing neurons, expanding the spaces, and increasing connections between neurons.

WHEN TO SEE A DOCTOR ABOUT MEMORY LOSS

If you have any of the following problems, in the absence of any other symptoms, you most likely do not need to consult a doctor:

- Forgetting names
- Misplacing keys, glasses, or other small items
- Not being able to find your car in a parking lot
- Not being able to remember items to shop for at the store
- Not being able to recognize someone in an unfamiliar setting

These symptoms do require medical investigation:

- Getting lost while driving a familiar route
- Completely forgetting important appointments
- Telling the same stories over and over to the same people during a short space of time (i.e., no short-term recall)
- Having periods of confusion over what time it is or where one is
- Being unable to manage a checkbook or take care of simple finances
- Experiencing a sudden or gradual change in personality
- Having difficulty with language (e.g., naming objects)
- Experiencing a sudden change in artistic or musical ability
- Undergoing a loss of memory which is disabling to the point that work is impossible or one's daily activity level is upset

Vernon Mark and Jeffrey Mark
Reversing Memory Loss

Traditionally, experts asserted that we only have a finite number of brain cells, and that after they are created, our brain cells don't reproduce anymore. However, more recently researchers have found that brain size and presumably the spaces, connections, or cells in it can be increased by an enriched physical environment. The question is whether or not nutrients and pharmaceuticals might also contribute to brain expansion. For example, David Krech, of the University of California at Berkeley, found that when rats were raised in more stimulating environments with mazes, swings, and slides to play with, they developed larger brains that weighed more. He found that the brains of stimulated rats had both more neurons and more complex neural networks, with more connections between cells. More recent studies showed that the same process seems to increase the brain size and the functioning of older rats.

Marian Diamond, a Berkeley scientist, found similar results when she provided elderly, two- and three-year-old rats with a more playful, stimulating environment, and gave them extra attention. The rats became more alert and intelligent than rats of the same age treated normally. She found their brains were bigger, particularly in the cerebral cortex area. Presumably the larger brains enabled the rats to learn and remember more. On top of this, these rats lived longer, too!

As Rosenfeld, author of *Prolongevity II*, observes, the results of Diamond's experiments suggest that "the more the brain is stimulated, even in advanced age, the more tissue there is to keep stimulating," and presumably the more the brain can do. The idea that brain cells can regenerate is supported by researchers who have found that new neurons continue to grow in fish and birds in adulthood. There seems to be a connection between learning, creating new memories, and brain growth. For example, in 1984, Fernando Nottebohm at Rockefeller University studied canaries and found a large growth of neurons in the area of the bird's forebrain that governs singing behavior after the fall season, when the birds learn the songs for the next breeding season. The birds lost about 40 percent of their old neurons after the preceding breeding season, presumably because of ordinary aging. Nottebohm's data suggest that the new cycle of learning new songs stimulated their brains to form new neurons.

There is mounting evidence that in humans the older brain can be changed to function better. Just imagine—as they might say in advertising—"Your new, improved brain!" University of Rochester researcher Paul Coleman did autopsies on healthy people sixty to ninety years old who had died of causes other than brain problems. He showed that the neuron's dendritic trees keep growing longer and continue to make new connections even in old age. Rosenfeld, who reviewed this research, points out that the idea of a limited number of brain cells that can't regenerate may be more folklore than fact.

If stimulating environments and new learning experiences can trigger the development of new brain cells, spaces, and connections in the brain, resulting in improved cognitive functioning, there is potential for promoting new brain cells, spaces, and connections with brain foods and smart drugs. As research accumulates, we are beginning to discover substances that can promote brain growth and improved brain functioning.

THINKING AND INTELLIGENCE

Memory is a key factor in thinking and intelligence. You must be able to recall words and ideas to be able to think about things, and better recall contributes to improved reasoning. But memory is not the only factor. Improved brain functioning can contribute to how well we think and to the other elements that make up intelligence.

Defining intelligence is complicated. Scientists are still debating whether intelligence tests accurately measure intelligence. Edwin Boring, a pragmatic scientist at Harvard, claimed back in 1923 that intelligence is "the capacity to do well in an intelligence test. Intelligence is what the tests test." But such a statement begs the question. There is no agreement on whether the tests in use adequately measure intelligence, since there are different views about what intelligence is and the components that make it up.

Certain abilities are widely considered to be elements of intelligence, most notably verbal agility, problem solving, and logical thinking skills. Other abilities considered to reflect intelligence include good relationship skills, manual dexterity, and the ability to create art or music. Scientists use the ability of the brain to react to a stimulus, as measured by the speed of dilation of the pupils when a light shines into the eyes, as an indicator of the speed of brain processing. This is in turn correlated to intellectual capability.

At one time, intelligence was thought to be fixed, based on what we were born with and how we were raised in early years. The classic Stanford-Binet I.Q. test given in elementary school reflected this thinking, for example. The theory was that the first test given in kindergarten revealed the individual's intelligence potential. The subsequent testing, usually in about the sixth grade, showed how the individual's intelligence stabilized by about age 12 or 13. The score was the person's intelligence quotient or I.Q. and was considered the most reliable predictor of what that person would be able to do mentally.

As the result of a growing body of research since the 1950s, experts now believe that mental functioning can be improved. One of the key studies has been the research of Marian Diamond, a neuroanatomist at the University of California. Besides showing that rats raised in an enriched environment had bigger brains and could remember more, her research also suggested that these big-brained rats could think better, too. They solve problems faster, which is considered a key component of general intelligence.

Diamond studied what happened to the brains of rats raised in three different conditions. She used rats because of the similarity between their brains and those of humans. The first condition was an *impoverished* environment, where a single rat was put in isolation in a regular-sized cage, a little like keeping a person in a prison isolation cell with virtually no stimulation apart from meals. The second condition was a *normal* environment, in which three rats were put together in a regular-sized laboratory cage, which provided food and water, but little else. Third was an *enriched* environment, in which three rats had a chance to get out of their cages for several minutes each day to experience a stimulating playground-like area with all sorts of toys and things to do, like exploring mazes. The results were the bigger brains noted earlier, with a thicker cerebral cortex. Not only were brain cells larger, but there were more of them. It seems that the brain can increase in size and capacity even at an advanced stage.

Although much of this research has been focused on memory and learning, these improvements in brain structure and functioning also contribute to other aspects of intelligence, such as problem solving. In her book *Enriching Heredity: The Impact of the Environment on the Anatomy of the Brain*, Diamond notes that other researchers have found that an enriched environment has resulted in research subjects being able to solve problems faster and more accurately.

Brain foods and smart drugs can also help to improve the number and size of neurons, size of the spaces, or number of connections, resulting in improved intelligence and thinking abilities. Enthusiasts believe that brain foods can help to reverse losses caused by age or other factors, such as illness or injury.

CHEMICAL INFLUENCES ON MEMORY, INTELLIGENCE, AND THINKING

The chemical mix in our brains plays a critical role in how well we remember and think. Another avenue to improve how our brain works is improving this chemical mix. The process is a little like putting additives into the gas for your car. The additives make your engine operate more efficiently and smoothly.

Chemical interplay in the brain is very complicated. For example, the hypothalamus in the brain plays an important role in maintaining the homeostasis or chemical equilibrium of the body. Among other things, this homeostasis regulates almost every activity in the physical system, including a fine balance between the various enzymes, hormones, and amines in the body. When the balance is optimally maintained, the chemical bath surrounding our neurons and the connections between them facilitates brain functioning.

The crucial role that this balance of brain chemicals plays in our state of mind is impressively demonstrated by the example of mental illness. Scientists now know that imbalances in the levels of key neurotransmitters including norepinephrine, dopamine, and serotonin are closely linked to mental disorders such as mania, schizophrenia, and depression. Perhaps it's no coincidence that people suffering from these conditions are sometimes called "unbalanced."

But as we age, this "homeostatic harmony" can become increasingly imbalanced. Unless we do something, there can be complications that interfere with how well our brains work. By the same token, injuries, illnesses, or even stress can interfere with optimal chemical balance, and lead to poorer functioning. As an analogy, consider what happens when we disrupt a juggler who has developed a careful routine to balance many balls in the air. The flow is disturbed, and the balls fall to the ground unless the juggler can manage to restore that harmonic balance.

Since there are so many chemicals that make up the harmonic mix, there are many ways in which our brain chemistry can go out of balance. Correspondingly, there are many ways in which we can intervene with brain foods and smart drugs to restore harmony.

One example of a decline in homeostasis that occurs with age is the increase of the enzyme monoamine oxidase (MAO) in the tissues. MAO is important because it performs the first step in the process of breaking down the amines formed in the body, including those that aid in the transmission of nerve-impulses through the brain. MAO "grabs" or binds to the amine molecules, beginning the chain of events whereby the amines are metabolized and eliminated from the body. MAO is like a molecular "Pac Man" roving through the system, gobbling up brain chemicals.

This is how MAO helps to maintain the balance of brain chemical levels of many important neurotransmitters, including serotonin, norepinephrine, and dopamine, which we discussed in an earlier chapter. For instance, if the body produces too much norepinephrine, a neurotransmitter that stimulates brain activity, the brain may overload. An example might be when one is absorbing so much new information so quickly that one gets a headache. MAO gets rid of the extra neurohormone, returning the brain and body back to its normal state of being in homeostatic balance.

The aging process interferes with the balance in this chemical process. Starting at about forty-five years of age, the levels of MAO in the body go up, destroying more than the usual amount of the amines. This disrupts the delicate balance of MAO with norepinephrine. Like a domino effect, the level of norepinephrine drops, which, in turn, depresses the level of activity in the brain and the central nervous system. The result is a decline in ability to think and remember, and sometimes to feelings of depression and a loss of interest in life. However, if one can inhibit the action of MAO, the amount of norepinephrine will go up, and along with it the level of brain activity.

IDENTIFY THE CAUSE OF MEMORY LOSS FIRST

Never just assume that if memory goes, it is gone forever. Literally scores of different conditions can result in a person's losing all or part of vital memory, conditions that are treatable and reversible. The important point to remember is that the problem or condition causing memory loss has to be identified. A rational course of treatment or prevention cannot begin until the problem has been precisely identified. If the problem is treatable, much can be done. And keep in mind, new information and better treatments are being developed every year.

Vernon Mark and Jeffrey Mark
Reversing Memory Loss

As scientists discover more about the various chains of chemical reactions in the brain, they learn how to use smart pharmaceuticals and nutrients to affect different enzymes, amines, and other chemicals in the process.

It sometimes appears possible to intervene on the molecular, atomic, or even the genetic level to improve the power of the brain. Denham Harman, a scientist at the University of Nebraska, suggests that one reason for mental deterioration with aging is that our bodies are attacked by certain molecules known as *free radicals*, which have a free or unpaired electron. According to Harman, free radicals are very unstable and dangerous to the functioning of the brain. Pairs of positive and negative particles are in balance and more stable. By contrast, free radicals are unstable, because they are missing an electron. Like single men cruising the bars looking for a date wherever they can find one, free radicals will steal an electron from any other molecule to create a complete pair again, thereby making themselves stable and whole. Unfortunately, the molecule that loses its electron to a free radical is damaged and may even be destroyed. It's like the married man who loses his wife to another man, and is rendered nonfunctional by the depression that results.

As attacks by free radicals increase over time with aging, more healthy molecules are damaged or destroyed. This contributes to the chronic degenerative diseases and decline in brain power. In fact, free radicals can create chain reactions of ever-increasing damage, because when a free radical steals an electron from another molecule, this produces another free radical, which goes on to seek out another molecule to steal from. So there's a kind of domino effect that contributes to further disrupting bodily and brain functioning on the cellular level.

Deterioration isn't inevitable, however. The process can be slowed or interrupted by substances created in the body called *antioxidants*. These substances have the ability to neutralize the destructive power of the free radicals.

Free radicals are produced within the body itself by the ordinary metabolic activities going on in the body. They are also created by environmental influences of all sorts, from ultraviolet light sources to x-rays, the chemical toxins around us, fats, oils, nuclear radiation, and smoking. In fact, it is difficult to avoid encountering things in our environment that promote production of free radicals. Even routine cooking contributes to development of free radicals. Exposure to air and heat step up the oxidation of fats; so cooking anything with fat creates free radicals.

Still, we do have some internal protections. Our body can neutralize most of the free radicals that are produced. One thing that helps is optimal nutrition. Certain enzymes and nutrients like vitamins C (ascorbic acid), E, B_2 (riboflavin), B_3 (niacinamide), and A (beta-carotene); minerals like selenium, zinc, copper, iron, and magnesium; amino acids like L-cysteine and L-methionine; and enzymes like glutathione peroxidase and superoxide dismutase counter the production of free radicals by promoting the body's own production of antioxidants. These vitamins and nutrients neutralize free radicals before they are able to attack other molecules, thereby stopping the chain reaction.

• • •

In this chapter we've looked at aspects of brain function that play a role in thinking and the formation of memory. We've seen how events that happen in the brain with aging interfere with these aspects of brain function. Drugs and nutrients that combat the mental effects of aging work by improving these brain functions or by preventing their impairment. It's easy to see how many of these same drugs and nutrients could improve brain function in people who aren't suffering from the mental effects of aging, helping such people to become "smarter."

4

BRAIN BOOSTERS: FOOD OR DRUGS?

"Smart drugs," "smart pills," "smart nutrients," "brain foods," and other terms referring to mind enhancers for memory, intelligence, and other mental functions are often used interchangeably. It is confusing. People wonder what the differences are between these substances.

As a general rule, nutrients include food substances, such as dosages of vitamins and minerals available in foods, and naturally occurring substances made by the body or in plants. Drugs, on the other hand, are synthesized chemicals. However, especially powerful or unusual combinations of vitamins, minerals, and nutrients, and various extracts, hormones, and enzymes have also been classified as drugs by the Food and Drug Administration (FDA).

The boundaries between foods and drugs can get very fuzzy. A nutritional substance that has numerous chemical additives may be considered to be a drug. Sometimes food substances are packaged as pills or capsules. Although the substance itself may be considered a nutrient, the way it is packaged and promoted might lead it to being classified as a drug by the FDA. From the point of view of brain food enthusiasts, such an FDA reclassification doesn't make the nutrient a drug in a true technical sense, even though the FDA decision makes it *legally* a drug and subject to FDA restrictions.

NUTRIENTS VERSUS DRUGS

Boundaries between nutrients and drugs are not hard and fast. There is considerable controversy over which is better for people to use. Some experts advise against taking any drugs and sticking to nutrients. They believe the nutrients are more natural, whereas drugs are synthetic substances. Other experts suggest that synthetics, whether classified as food supplements, nutrients, or drugs, are less expensive, purer, and better.

The "natural versus synthetic" debate is discussed at length in *Life Extension*, by Durk Pearson and Sandy Shaw, who discredit the claims of the pure naturalists as myth, because "all foods, vitamins, and nutrients, and all the other substances of life, are chemicals." Accordingly, whether a particular chemical compound is produced within one's own body or obtained from external sources, such as a food supplement or pill, it is still the same chemical. A molecule of vitamin C is still a molecule of vitamin C, for example, whether it is made as a synthetic in a chemical factory, or is made naturally by a plant's biochemical factory. Paraphrasing Gertrude Stein's "A rose is a rose is a rose," Pearson and Shaw say, "A vitamin C is a vitamin C is a vitamin C."

Pearson and Shaw point out that some synthetically made substances may actually be more beneficial to the individual than a naturally occurring substance, because it is purer, whereas some natural vitamin extracts have impurities with undesirable properties. For example, there may be pollen impurities that some people are allergic to in natural vitamin C, whereas synthetic vitamin C has no such impurities.

Sometimes a synthetic vitamin may be more biologically usable by the body, because the natural substance may be in a form that is hard for the body to use. In the natural state certain types of vitamin C have membrane-binding factors that hold it in position so that the plant from which it is extracted can germinate, for example. Before such vitamin C can be used in the human body, the membrane structures must be broken down. By contrast, the body doesn't have to break down synthetic vitamin C before using it. Pearson and Shaw argue that synthetic vitamins can be preferable because they are much less expensive than natural vitamins, which can be a significant factor for people taking large quantities of vitamins.

TOXICITY AND POTENCY

One noteworthy aspect of the nootropics and some of the other "intelligence enhancers" is that several of these compounds apparently feature multiple vectors of pharmacological action. Among these chemicals, we find at least two products used . . . in treating depression as well as age-related syndromes, specifically Alzheimer's and Parkinson's disease. Different compounds falling under this rubric have also been credited with immune-enhancing, life-extending, and detoxifying properties. Some nootropics and other similarly employed drugs have low— if even measurable—toxicity, and a few even show "healthy side effects" such as increasing the flow of oxygen and nutrients to nervous tissue. For example, one official of the Food and Drug Administration recently claimed that the toxicity of piracetam is so low that this compound could, in principle, have no significant action—a fallacy based on a pharmacological axiom long rendered obsolete by observations of the relationship between the potency, effects, and as yet unestablished toxicity of LSD. Such phenomena are beginning to blur the boundary between drugs—once widely understood as "poisons" of medicinal value in subtoxic doses—and nutrients.

Dan Joy
from the Introduction to the *Psychedelic Encyclopedia*,
3rd edition, by Peter Stafford

From this perspective, such chemical substances, whether naturally produced or synthetic, are still nutrients or nutrient supplements, since they occur naturally in the body or in plants or can be synthesized

FDA DEFINES SMART DRUGS

The term smart drugs is applied to various products, many of which are actually nutrients—amino acids, vitamins, or other food substances such as choline, which is derived from lecithin—as well as herbs and certain unapproved drugs and prescription drugs. Powdered nutrient supplements such as the amino acids phenylalanine and alanine, as well as choline, are being widely promoted as "cognitive enhancers" and in some cases mixed with beverages and sold at "health bars" as "smart drinks."

Proponents claim the products stimulate mental function, improve performance, attention and concentration, and increase cognition and intelligence. Smart drugs are often purchased through off-shore or overseas pharmacies, foreign mail-order firms and health-food outlets in the United States. Occasionally they are obtained fraudulently through physicians' prescriptions or imported for personal use.

While the FDA is concerned about the safety of the food-based products such as amino acids and vitamins, those that are prescription drugs pose even greater risks. The drugs are frequently imported from areas outside FDA jurisdiction and often do not meet quality-control standards commonly accepted in this country and enforced by the FDA. The agency announced an import alert directed at unapproved mail-order drugs sold by off-shore companies. Included were some drugs promoted as smart drugs.

FDA Talk Paper

as a chemical twin. Purists, however, may regard such substances (especially if they are taken in large quantities) as a drug. For example, in *Secrets of Life Extension,* John Mann observes "any vitamin, mineral, or other nutritional factor may be regarded as an anti-aging drug" because, when taken in large-enough doses, "they have protective and

therapeutic properties, distinct from their usual nutritional functions."
From this perspective, when a nutritional supplement is taken in huge
doses, it becomes a drug, because it is used not just to nourish, but also
to prevent damage or improve bodily and mental functioning.

Thus, the line between smart foods and smart drugs can be very
fuzzy, indeed. It seems that simply increased quantities turn nutrients
that nourish into drugs that protect and improve. Mann gives several
examples of how vitamins can protect the body from damage and
improve functioning. Such protective or improved functioning can, in
turn, influence how the brain works. For example, Mann notes that
vitamin D can serve as an anti-stress agent, because it maintains good
amounts of calcium, which has a calming effect in the blood. B vitamins— especially vitamin B_6 (pyridoxine), PABA (para-aminobenzoic
acid), vitamin B_2 (riboflavin), vitamin B_3 (niacin), and vitamin B_{12}
(cobalamine)—can also function as anti-stress factors. Any vitamin
that reduces stress, Mann argues, can contribute to mental functioning,
since stress disrupts concentration, clear thinking, and memory.

Mann also suggests that minerals, when taken in large quantities,
act as drugs. Some of these minerals—for example, calcium and
magnesium—are normally present in the body in fairly large quantities;
others are trace minerals, normally present in very small quantities,
such as molybdenum, vanadium, and cobalt. But often, extra quantities
of certain common or trace minerals will improve bodily or mental
functioning. For example, the minerals magnesium, potassium, and
calcium are helpful in reducing stress and keeping the body in balance.
Chromium, iron, and molybdenum appear to slow down aging, according to Mann's research.

HERBS

Classifying herbs, which are plants used for both their nutritional
value and their therapeutic or medicinal properties, opens up the same
sort of controversy. Herbs are commonly used by chopping up the
leaves, roots, and bark into a powder or brewing them into a tea. Herbs
are foods when used to flavor a food dish, such as a soup, salad, or

vegetable dish. However, at other times, it may not be clear whether herbs should be considered a food or a drug, for example when herbs are brewed into a tea. Is the tea just a drink, or might it be taken for medicinal purposes, making it perhaps a drug? Some herbs may be clearly used for a therapeutic or medical purpose, as when concentrated herb extract is used or herb salve is applied to the forehead to treat a headache.

HERBS AND DRUGS COMPARED

Although herbs have therapeutic properties, they should not be thought of or classified as drugs. Herbs contain a mixture of naturally occurring substances that often possess a number of therapeutic effects. Drugs are generally refined, purified, and concentrated forms of a single substance that is designed to have a single therapeutic effect. Herbs are generally more gentle and tonic-like, whereas drugs are strong, selective in their effects, and may have toxic side effects.

Ross Pelton
Mind Foods and Smart Pills

Many experts define herbs used for therapeutic purposes as drugs. From their perspective, it is the intended use of the herb that determines its classification.

In short, one's point of view is important in determining when vitamins, minerals, and herbs are considered foods or drugs. In some situations, the FDA may define a substance as a drug. For the purposes of this book, the vitamins, minerals, and herbs are being grouped together as nutrients. However, depending on the amount used or the purpose for which they are used, they may be considered drugs by some people.

A good example of how something normally used as a food can be turned into a drug is given by the research that New York University professor Harry Demopoulis did with vitamins C and E. Usually, these vitamins would be considered nutrients, since they are a normal, naturally occurring substance in many foods, and are commonly used as dietary supplements. When Demopoulis was researching free radicals, the damage they do to cells, and methods to overcome this damage, he discovered that when vitamins C and E are used together, they improve each other's effectiveness in combating cell destruction by free radicals. Demopoulis theorized that each of the vitamins would go after a particular free-radical target and counter its damage, although there might be some overlap. Thus, if vitamin C missed a particular radical, vitamin E might go after that radical, and vice versa. An analogy might be two cops in a melée deciding to apprehend different drunken fighters, though occasionally they might work together to take on a particularly difficult antagonist. Demopoulis concluded that vitamins as antitoxidants could act as important protective substances. He recommended that they should be taken in relatively high doses and in combination with one another to increase the chances of preventing or reducing the damage of free radicals. In addition to vitamins C and E, Demopoulis believes that many of the B vitamins, taken in megadoses, more than 30 times the normally suggested RDA (Recommended Daily Allowance), can also be beneficial. Given the high doses and the therapeutic purpose, vitamins used in this way might be considered a drug.

Packaging and dosage also affect a substance's classification. For example, if a vitamin is packaged as a regular nutritional substance, it might be prepared in capsules or with relatively small dosages, around the amount commonly taken or suggested by RDA guidelines. People wanting to use it therapeutically, more as a drug than as a nutrient, can take several capsules; but because the substance is packaged for normal nutritional use, it would still remain classified as a nutrient. However, if the substance is prepared to provide individual megadoses, designed for specific therapeutic use, then it might be viewed as a drug.

Because distinctions are not normally made or are unclear in the literature, in this book, vitamins will be classified as nutrients, regardless of the dosage or purpose. On the other hand, novel chemical combinations that are used for cognitive enhancement or other therapeutic purposes will be classified as drugs. Finally, special therapeutic treatments that are clearly medical in nature will be discussed as drugs. For example, cell therapy is an anti-aging treatment that seeks to reverse the aging process's effect on the body, including symptoms of mental decline. Cell therapy involves injecting the patient with a solution made from fresh, living cells from the organs of a sheep fetus, removed from its mother one month before it is supposed to be born. Although the fetuses of other animals could be used, practitioners using this process prefer sheep because of their high resistance to disease. Reportedly this process has been very effective and has been used successfully on more than 10,000 people in Europe, including some very well-known people, such as famous actors, authors, artists, politicians, and even Pope Pius XII. In the U.S. this therapy is not allowed by the FDA, and people are not allowed to import freeze-dried sheep fetus cells. Treatments of this sort that have a therapeutic impact on mental functioning will be mentioned, even though they are not approved by the FDA for use in the United States. If their use is therapeutic they will be classified along with the drugs.

However, although these different substances will be discussed in separate categories in the following chapters, it should be emphasized that the distinctions are often arbitrary. There is often no clear agreement about when something should be considered a nutrient or when it is a drug. Moreover, many nutrients and drugs, however they are defined, may be used for similar purposes to produce certain chemical changes or specific effects in the body or mind. Thus, though nutrients and drugs will be distinguished for purposes of classifying and discussing different types of substances and their effects in subsequent chapters, it is important to realize that either or both may be used singly or in combination to produce desired changes.

5

THE BUSINESS OF SMART DRUGS AND NUTRIENTS

The popularity of brain foods and smart drinks is infectious; so it's not too surprising that they have become big business. The sale of brain-boosting drugs, nutrients, and herbs as well as of magazines, books, lectures, and tapes that support their promotion, is soaring. Sales are both above and below ground. According to the *Washington Drug Newsletter* between 1987 and 1992, smugglers brought more than 15 tons of smart drugs into the U.S. without FDA approval.

SALES THROUGH THE DRUG AND PHARMACEUTICAL INDUSTRY

Until the early 1990s, cognitive-enhancing drugs were on the fringes of the established pharmaceutical industry, because most had not been approved for sale in the United States. However, many were selling briskly in Europe and could be obtained by Americans by mail order through foreign sources. At the same time, many brain-boosting nutrients started to come under the scrutiny of the FDA with an emphasis on scheduling them as actual "drugs."

The potential of cognitive-enhancing drugs for future sales in the pharmaceutical industry is tremendous. Christina Hauer, a financial analyst writing in *Barron's*, a leading financial weekly, pointed out that the legal drug business worldwide is about $150 billion per year. A few super pharmaceutical companies dominate the industry: Glaxo, Merck, Pfizer, Bristol-Myers, Squibb, Smithkline, and Syntex. Six of these seven pharmaceutical giants are in the United States. Some people call them the "Seven Sisters of Pharmaceuticals"—like the seven major oil companies—referring to the Pleiades, a group of seven stars in the constellation Taurus called the Seven Sisters by the ancient Greeks. To give you a measure of their size: Merck and Glaxo spend more than $1 billion a year on R&D and capital expenditures.

Even though smart drugs have gained considerable mainstream support in Europe, the power of the U.S. drug industry to determine the development and availability of future smart drugs is tremendous. As Hauer observes, "In terms of technological leadership, there are few industries where we are so firmly established as Number One as the pharmaceutical industry." There was a flow of scientific talent into the pharmaceutical and biotech industry during the 1980s that gave the U.S. pharmaceutical industry substantial control over the future of the smart-drugs phenomenon."

Traditionally, the policy of the pharmaceutical industry has been to keep most smart drugs out of the country, to limit the legal application of these drugs to specific medical purposes, such as the treatment of Alzheimer's disease, and to push for restrictions on nutrients by classifying them as drugs. There is much speculation that their underlying motive was to protect their domination of the industry by preventing new products from being developed by individuals and outside companies. Given the size and growing power of the industry, the potential for even bigger sales of smart drugs is tremendous should established pharmaceutical companies jump on the bandwagon. In the process, the small entrepreneurial companies that created the industry will be pushed out.

A key reason for the recent growth of the smart-drugs market is the aging of the baby-boomer generation and its entrance into middle age. In the early 1990s, the ages of the baby-boomers ranged from 35 to 50, and they accounted for about 40 percent of the U.S. population. It's in this age range that people begin to manifest chronic ailments associated with aging. Boomers have been characterized by an obsession with youth: it was the baby-boomers who brought us the psychedelic '60s and its drug-friendly ideology; so it's not too surprising that, as they notice lapses in memory and a decline in mental alertness, boomers should be attracted to the idea of popping a pill to make one smarter.

The potential market share for smart drugs is substantial. Financial analysts estimate that the U.S. market for smart pills will be more than $1 billion per year. This could be a conservative figure, considering that many Americans are buying smart drugs outside the U.S. and cognitive-enhancing nutrients outside regular pharmaceutical channels. If one adds sales of smart products by smart bars and cafés at rave parties, at health-food stores, and at concessions at informal events like county fairs and street festivals, along with the sales through network and multilevel marketing channels, the size of the market could be substantially larger than the billion-dollar estimate.

The possibilities for sales are just beginning because of the growing armies of people taking smart drugs and nutrients. For example, in a 1991 *USA Today* article, smart-drugs expert John Morgenthaler estimated about 100,000 people in the U.S. were taking smart drugs, up from about zero ten years before. Given this growth rate, the numbers are probably in the hundreds of thousands, and growing every day, as more people learn about the benefits of smart drugs and discover ways to obtain them. In turn, such numbers translate into growing profits for those companies making such drugs, whether in the pharmaceutical mainstream or outside it.

MARKETING SMART DRUGS AND NUTRIENTS THROUGH MULTILEVEL MARKETING

Smart nutrients, herbs, and drink preparations have been snatched up by multilevel marketing companies, where a network of salespeople sell directly to consumers. The multilevel marketing (MLM) industry, pioneered by Amway and Shaklee in the 1950s and 1960s, has become a $35 billion industry worldwide, with sales of $9 to 10 billion in the

U.S., according to Gini Graham Scott, author of *Success in Multi-Level Marketing.* It's an approach that markets products not available in stores directly to the consumer, usually in an informal setting. Simultaneously, they recruit others to sell and then get a commission from their sales. Those people, in turn, recruit new salespeople. It takes on a pyramid structure, with people at each level selling, and commissions from lower-level sales flowing upward to those above. With a good product line, good management, and people who are actively selling the products to customers, MLM has a tremendous potential to generate an explosive growth with high profits for everyone. The potential arises largely from the override system, in which salespeople get commissions not only on what they sell, but also on the sales of the people they recruit and the people these people recruit and so on. Some of the most successful distributors in MLM systems earn hundreds of thousands of dollars a year. During times of economic doldrums, such as in the early 1990s, MLM companies tend to grow especially fast, as out-of-work and underemployed people look to MLM as a chance to achieve the "American dream" of super-success and financial freedom through hard work.

Entrepreneurs jumped on the opportunities presented by the brain-boosting boom to develop new products and set up MLM companies to promote them. Take the story of Jerry Rubin. In the 1960s Rubin was a yippie revolutionary, who led radicals in confrontations with the system and earned fame for his cliché, "Don't trust anyone over 30." In the 1970s, he was one of the pioneers of the human-potential movement. In the 1980s, he went into business as a stockbroker and founded a number of high-profile networking business clubs for "yuppies." In the 1990s, he became one of the most successful and high-profile distributors in an MLM company founded by three distributors of Herbalife International known as Omnitrition International of Carrollton, Texas, which sold vitamin drinks. Early in 1992 Rubin boasted 10,000 distributors that he called "individual entrepreneurs" who generated $15 million a year in sales. Of this attractive pie, Rubin earned $600,000, less expenses.

To support its growing sales network, Omnitrition provided commercial or "slick" sales literature, including a monthly video magazine, *Omnivision*, which brought its salespeople the latest information on new products, training updates, retailing tips, and life-style success stories. A monthly newsletter, *Omni News*, highlighted the latest success stories of distributors all over the country, many of whom went from financial disasters to making thousands of dollars each month, along with tips for how to make more money, and data on company bonus and incentive plans. They provided product literature and samples designed to whet people's appetite.

The names of product lines are very trendy. Pearson and Shaw's product line is called Designer Mind Foods™. Individual products include: *Wow!™*, which is a nutritional beverage mix; *Go For It!™*, a caffeine-free nutrient supplement; and *Focus™*, a nutritional beverage mix providing "nutrients for the brain." *Memory Fuel™*, described as a Mental Fitness™ Drink mix, contains a natural fruit-flavored choline brain food. Other enticing products are Earth Girl's "Psuper Psonic Psybertonic" claimed to increase mental capacity and fine-tune focusing powers, and "Energy ElickSure" claimed to invigorate the body, and provide a natural energetic feeling and stimulation without caffeine and the tired coffee crash.

As smart products grow in popularity, they can be expected to move into the mainstream with other multilevel and direct-sales companies actively promoting them. It is likely that the large, established health-oriented MLM companies specializing in dietary and nutritional supplements, such as Herbalife, Neo-Life, BodyWise, Sunrider, and Lite & Rite, will bring out their own smart-product lines.

BUYING SMART PRODUCTS BY MAIL

Since many smart products have not yet been approved for use in the U.S., smart products purchased from foreign sources have become a big mail-order business. Many people purchase brain boosters from suppliers in Mexico, Europe, and the Cayman Islands.

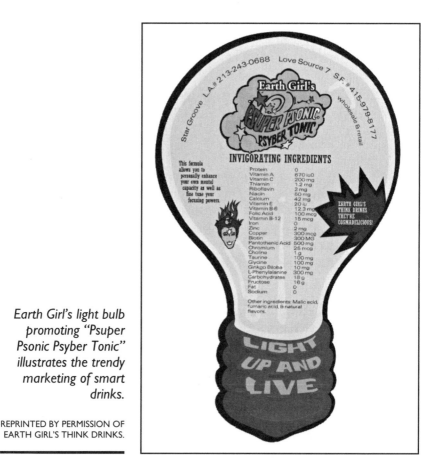

Earth Girl's light bulb promoting "Psuper Psonic Psyber Tonic" illustrates the trendy marketing of smart drinks.

REPRINTED BY PERMISSION OF EARTH GIRL'S THINK DRINKS.

An early issue of *Smart Drug News* pointed out that many smart drugs are available "over-the-counter in Mexico." All one needed to do was to get to the border, walk across, take a taxi to the nearest pharmacy, and buy the drugs one wants. However, while the border patrol will allow people to bring back a "reasonable" quantity of most drugs—approximately a three-month supply—they cautioned that drugs that "are controlled in the United States will probably be confiscated." The magazine recommended getting a prescription from a sympathetic U.S. doctor for extra protection. While a "script" isn't needed to purchase smart drugs in Mexico, it can help reduce the possibility of problems at the border.

For those who don't travel, there are always the mails. Interlab is a mail-order pharmacy that was created in response to a FDA ruling that allowed people in the U.S. to import a three-month personal supply of drugs as long as they are considered safe in the country from which ordered. This ruling was made because of pressure from AIDS political-action groups, who argued that they were being prevented from obtaining potentially life-saving substances. In addition to drugs believed to be life-saving for AIDS sufferers, Interlab carries a variety of cognitive-enhancement and life-extension drugs not available in the U.S. No prescription is necessary for purchase. However, in the spring of 1992, access to foreign drugs for personal use became clouded as the FDA threatened another crackdown.

In January 1992, FDA field officers were instructed in an "Import Alert" to automatically detain all imported drugs entering the United States from six overseas companies, including InHome Health Services and Interlab. This "embargo" covers non-FDA approved drugs like piracetam and Lucidril, and foreign versions of drugs approved in the U.S., like hydergine and vasopressin. Americans ordering drugs such as vasopressin from Interlab, for example, received notices from the FDA that after January all orders would be confiscated. However, a loophole remained open. Previously the FDA allowed entry of "personal-use" quantities, which is a three-month supply or less, of certain smart drugs not approved for use in the U.S. "provided that the drugs do not pose unreasonable safety risks, that their use is not promoted in the United States, and that they are for serious conditions for which there is not satisfactory treatment available in this country." However, in January 1992 the FDA began closing this loophole, and issued new rules that use of the drug had to be supervised by a physician, and that the person had to be suffering a life-threatening or debilitating illness. In other words, a physician's letter stating that one is under medical supervision and explaining what debilitating illness the drug is needed for may allow shipments through, but there is no guarantee.

The Mail Order Pharmacy in Lighthouse Point, Florida, provides another avenue for obtaining smart drugs. With a doctor's prescription,

Life Extension Foundation members can order smart drugs that have been approved for use in the United States. Of course, the problem is that most doctors know little about cognitive enhancement and life extension; so the first hurtle is finding a knowledgeable doctor. The American College of Advancement in Medicine (ACAM) in Laguna Hills, California, maintains a directory of physicians knowledgeable in life extension. Dr. Ward Dean suggests that readers can call them for names of physicians in their area. The Life Extension Foundation in Ft. Lauderdale, Florida, publishes *The Directory of Life Extension Doctors*, which is reprinted here in Appendix A. Foundation members receive a copy of the latest updated *Directory* with their membership. The *Directory* lists doctors throughout the United States and in many foreign countries, including Australia, Belgium, Brazil, Canada, Denmark, the Dominican Republic, Egypt, England, France, West Germany, Indonesia, Mexico, the Netherlands, New Zealand, Puerto Rico, the Philippines, Spain, Switzerland, Taiwan, and the West Indies. Doctors are selected for inclusion in the *Directory* in terms of their knowledge of nutrition, preventive medicine, and life extension. As part of a life-extension and optimal health-care program, a doctor might prescribe anti-aging drugs, including smart drugs. Prescriptions can be mailed or faxed to The Mail Order Pharmacy. Alternatively, doctors can call in prescriptions directly.

Each drug received from The Mail Order Pharmacy is accompanied by a Drug Information Sheet that describes the potential side effects and contraindications of the drug ordered. The service is specialized. The pharmacist, Dr. Alan Zimmer, maintains a file on each patient. Whenever a drug is ordered, Dr. Zimmer reviews the file to guard against drug interactions. Additionally, he is available by phone for consultation about one's life-extension program.

Deprenyl and THA (Tacrine or Cognex) are available by mail through the Alzheimer's Buyer's Club in Costa Rica. Deprenyl has been approved in the U.S. for the treatment of Parkinson's dwisease, and has shown promise as a means of boosting sex drive, relieving depression, and slowing the aging process, but such uses have not been approved by the FDA. Research by Dr. William Summers has shown that a combination of THA and lecithin improves recent memory and the daily-living activities associated with improved short-term memory in Alzheimer's patients. But, until recently, the FDA has refused to approve THA therapy for Alzheimer's disease. In response, relatives of patients suffering from Alzheimer's established a newsletter called *The Caregiver* and the Alzheimer's Buyer's Club. According to Dr. Ward Dean, THA has now been approved. He warns that THA is potentially hepatotoxic (toxic to the liver) and should never be used without a physician's supervision. Dr. Dean emphatically emphasizes that THA should not be used as a "smart drug" except in Alzheimer's disease.

Longevity Plus is a Longevity Buyer's Club in Czechoslovakia that supplies most of the popular smart drugs. A disclaimer on their order form states: "We are unable to enter into personal correspondence or offer any medical advice. Please ensure you are complying with your own country's laws; goods are shipped at buyer's risk." Sending one's money off to a company that refuses correspondence and states that goods are shipped at the buyer's risk is, indeed, worrisome. However, correspondence of any sort can be seen as promotion and distribution of unapproved drugs, which is illegal under FDA regulations.

In the U.S., mail-order companies can't sell drugs; so they market only smart nutritional supplements. Life Extension International in Florida publishes *The Directory of Life Extension Nutrients and Drugs,* which is a directory of products legal in the United States, provided free to members of the Life Extension Foundation. It lists a large selection of nutrients and vitamins. Each product is explained in substantial detail, including what it is, such as being an antioxidant, for example, and what effects its use has on the body, such as increasing endurance. Products can be ordered by phone. Smart Products in San Francisco has a more commercial approach. They promote a variety of health products and nutrients with snappy names suggesting high energy and brain enhancement, including several developed by Sandy Shaw and Durk Pearson.

There are enticing futuristic ads in magazines like *Mondo 2000* with headlines featuring neologisms like: "Explore Exotropic Futopia— Calling All Neuronauts?" and an attractive hairless woman with electrifying currents emanating from her third eye through the brain is the central design element. The ad promotes four popular Pearson and Shaw Designer Mind Foods™ available by mail order from Life Services Supplements, and offers distributorships, which are referred to as "the best financial opportunity of the '90s."

Sometimes multilevel-like incentives are provided by mail-order services, such as that provided by Nutritional Engineering, Ltd., which markets drugs from the Cayman Islands in the British West Indies. The

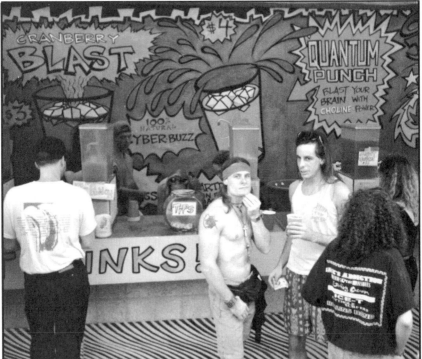

MARK RENNIE

SMART BARS FOR HIRE: Smart Products has exposed over 750,000 alternative music fans to the "intelligent alternative" by taking its "SMARTBAR™" on the road with the LOLLAPALOOZA tour. Traveling to over thirty cities, the SMARTBAR™ has served its delicious amino-acid and vitamin cocktails to fans and bands alike. Smart Products has also been heavily featured in tour coverage on MTV and in Rolling Stone, Newsweek, *and* Time *magazines, creating brand-name recognition and product demand among more than 7 million music fans.*

company features a variety of Gerovital formulations called "Vitacel," developed by Dr. Robert Koch, plus some vitamin and nutrient mixtures. To make the actual purchases, individuals must order from the company in the British West Indies. For those interested in participating in the MLM structure, which includes commissions for referrals down five levels for a 50 percent payout, there is a local address for getting product literature in Concord, California. Although much of the marketing effort may be conducted in the U.S., payouts to reward referrals are issued from a Cayman bank, with a $3 service charge deducted.

Such firms are just the tip of a growing iceberg. As the demand for brain boosters grows, more companies are springing up in the U.S. and abroad to fill the demand. The FDA is increasingly keeping a watchful eye on these companies and the claims that their products improve mental functioning. There is a kind of dance going on between entrepreneurs and the FDA, as the entrepreneurs try to respond to the demand and parry the latest moves of the FDA, while the FDA tries to crack down. By the summer of 1992 many smart-product entrepreneurs were running scared and were combining forces to fight back.

THE SMART-PRODUCTS BUSINESS AND THE RAVE SCENE

Finally, there is a growing market for the smart products at the rave scene. This is a somewhat less organized, more informal entrepreneurial business run by ravers who have adopted with-it business names for their enterprise. Typical of this group of high-tech hippie types called "cyberpunks" is an early smart-drinks business called "Get Smart Think Drinks." Wearing day-glo futuristic clothing, they mixed up their smart drinks in blenders, under the leadership of Earth Girl, its 21-year-old proprietor and bartender. Another enterprise found at many Toon Town raves is "The Nutrient Café" operated by Chris Beaumont. Many of these bars feature drinks made from Pearson and Shaw products; others develop their own secret formulas.

Such groups do the rave circuit with smart bars and nutrient cafés that average $3 to $4 a drink, and can pull in from about $1,000 gross a night at the smaller raves, with perhaps 200 to 300 people, to about $5,000 at the bigger raves, such as Toon Town's gala New Year's Eve bashes.

Such efforts are relatively small scale and unorganized in the larger scheme of smart-products marketing. People running the smart bars are not as high-powered and ambitious as those in the MLM and mail-order enterprises. Smart-bar proprietors are mostly 18- to 30-year-old rave fans, who are also fans of these products and take them themselves. Many of the raves are haphazard, underground adventures, which shift locations from night to night. Characteristic of the authentic rave is that its promoters do not announce where the rave will be until the afternoon of the event. People have to go to a selected location to get a ticket with a map letting them know where the rave will be. They are often held at places like a large field or a ranch fifty miles outside a major city such as San Francisco or in underground, questionable (by non-raver standards) locations like old warehouses and ghetto-area storefronts. For instance, participants going to a San Francisco Bay Area rave were given maps to an armory in Pittsburg, California, about forty miles away. On another night, the map led to a second floor of a South of Market warehouse near flophouse hotels, pawnshops, and liquor stores, where ravers took a freight elevator up to a long dark crowded room that looked like it usually stacked boxes, not people. On the face of it, raves are definitely not the sort of scene that would pull big business.

The rave movement is definitely growing, with increasing numbers of events being organized each week. Artfully colored announcements, reminiscent of the '60s' concert handbills, telling of upcoming raves, are handed out at previous ones and available at cyberpunk record and clothing stores. With several raves a week in several major U.S. and U.K. cities, and with about 1,000 ravers per rave, there are perhaps 10,000 ravers per city, maybe 50,000 to 100,000 nationally, and growing. The smart products businesses at raves are growing, too. Figure about $5,000 gross per rave, maybe $50,000 per weekend per city, maybe $250,000 to $500,000 nationally: that translates into about $1.2 to $2.5 million a year. The rave-scene sales are a drop in the bucket, compared to the other ways of marketing the smart products.

But the growing visibility of raves in the press with the increased interest in the rave smart bars helps the sale of brain boosters through other channels.

6

THE WAR OVER VITAMINS

With growing interest in brain boosters came increased concern about public welfare. In the early 1990s, Congress pushed the FDA to take a closer look at policies governing medical devices, pharmaceuticals, foods, and nutrients available to the public. The result was a tightening of requirements on what products were permitted and what companies were allowed to say about product benefits. There were several FDA enforcement raids on manufacturers, pharmacies, mail-order distributors, and doctors involved in the business.

Advocates responded by organizing grass-roots efforts to combat FDA policies. As part of this effort, in the Fall of 1992, Health Freedom publications issued a book titled *Stop the FDA*, edited by John Morgenthaler and Steven Fowkes. This book gathers together essays, articles, and research papers by journalists, doctors, health practitioners, and other advocates to form a fervent case against the FDA. Its viewpoint is epitomized by the Nobel-prize winning economist Milton Friedman's statement, "Any increase in the FDA's authority over anything is a clear and present danger to the nation's health."

In 1976 Congress passed the Proxmire Amendment. In part, the Amendment said that food, including dietary supplements, could not be reclassified as drugs solely because they exceed FDA-recommended levels of potency. From 1976 until 1990, vitamins and supplements received much less federal oversight than did other drugs and foods.

Nonetheless, people assumed that products in health-food stores had been subjected to the same safety standards as other foods sold in the U.S. Consumers didn't realize that many nutritional supplements had been developed by entrepreneurial chemists, and had not been subjected to any consumer safety standards. Containers didn't carry a list of side effects or toxicities, and were not child-proof or tamper-resistant. Things got so loose that salesmen were making drug-like therapeutic claims that critics characterized as being no better than nineteenth-century claims for "snake oil." People were encouraged to use vitamins as a quick fix for poor eating habits and as a substitute for medical treatment.

THE NUTRITIONAL LABELING AND EDUCATION ACT (NLEA)

In December 1990, Dr. David Kessler, who was only 39 years old, took over command of the FDA as commissioner. His credentials were impressive. Trained as a physician, Kessler also held an MBA and a law degree. He was the medical director of the hospital at Albert Einstein College of Medicine in the Bronx, and taught food and drug law at the Columbia University School of Law. Kessler didn't appear to be a typical bureaucrat. He co-authored John Hopkins University Press's book *Caring for the Elderly: Reshaping Health Policy.* While serving as Albert Einstein Hospital's medical director, he set aside time each week to see sick children in one of New York's municipal emergency rooms. Quickly he came to be called "the activist commissioner" by some.

In a watershed incident, more than thirty people died and hundreds suffered blood disorders linked to a contaminated batch of the amino acid tryptophan, which was readily available in health-food stores and used regularly by thousands of trusting Americans. The FDA subsequently banned the distribution and sale of tryptophan. Further controversy was generated by the fact that the ban remained in effect even though the Centers for Disease Control successfully linked all cases of the blood problem to a small number of contaminated batches manufactured by a company in Japan.

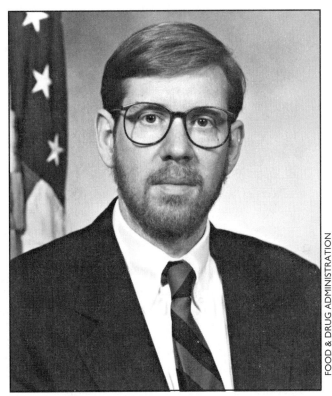

Dr. David Kessler, Commissioner of the FDA, took initiatives to revamp regulatory policy. In this context, David Kessler rose to the challenge and redirected the FDA with bold policy initiatives designed to protect the public from what he perceived to be potential risk.

FOOD & DRUG ADMINISTRATION

The public was again shaken by the revelation that breast implants were, in fact, dangerous. Believing they were safe, thousands of women underwent surgical breast implants. When problems occurred years later, the manufacturer, DOW Chemicals, admitted it had known there were risks when it released the implants to the market.

Congress passed the NLEA (Nutritional Labeling and Education Act) in 1990, and it was signed into law by President Bush in 1991. The stated goal was to provide the American public with better information on the health benefits of food, including supplements, and to protect Americans from unwarranted health claims. The Act instructed the FDA to develop guidelines for what kinds of information would be required or permitted on food products.

TOTALITARIAN TACTICS

The Food and Drug Administration . . . has carried out an unprecedented and systematic campaign to control the food, vitamin, nutrient, and medical decisions of United States citizens. To some readers—those on the receiving end of FDA enforcement actions—the previous sentence is an understatement. Picture instead: black leather boots kicking down doors; automatic weapons drawn and aimed at doctors, nurses, patients, business owners, employees, and customers; repeated raids intended to discourage co-operation with the press; self-serving press conferences with career-minded bureaucrats congratulating their own actions—all this smacks of totalitarian political tactics. To many Americans, these scenes are completely unbelievable. This isn't the "freedom and opportunity" that we were taught about America in school. This isn't what we read in the Constitution. This isn't what our forefathers envisioned when they created the government for which we vote.

John Morgenthaler and Steven Wm. Fowkes
Stop the FDA

As a step in developing the guidelines required by NLEA, Kessler convened a Dietary Supplement Task Force. The Task Force recommended that many common health claims, such as describing the benefits of high fiber, antioxidants, and unsaturated fatty acids, not be permitted on food products including supplements. This was called "labeling." Because these benefits had not been "proven" under the FDA's strict requirements, these claims couldn't be made on the label or product literature. Second, they urged that the Recommended Daily Allowance (RDA) for vitamins, minerals, and other nutrients be replaced with the Reference Daily Intake (RDI), which should be considerably *lower* than the RDA. The rationale behind the reduction was that the RDAs were established during World War II for on-duty soldiers.

However, since the War it had been used as a single standard for all people. They argued that a young man obviously needs more vitamins and nutrients than the rest of the population. As a result, recommended levels were higher than needed for most people. They recommended that on food labels, the RDI would be listed as a Daily Value (DV). They suggested moving away from "recommending" specific amounts of vitamins and minerals. Clarifying this, Edward Scarbrough, director of the FDA Office of Nutrition and Food Services Labels, said that the information on the label was to be a reference, and the thrust was for consumers to find out their own recommended amounts. The new orientation was to rely on a lot of consumer education.

However, the Task Force did go on to recommend restrictions on the use of educational material in the promotion of dietary supplements, even when written by a third party, and not specific to any product.

Task Force members turned to the regulation model used by the Drug Enforcement Agency (DEA) to enforce federal drug law. Drugs like cocaine and LSD are assigned *schedules* by the DEA depending on the level of restriction. Following this model, the Task Force proposed a three-category system of classification. To Category 1 would be assigned multivitamins and multiminerals with potencies no higher than those found in natural foods. For example, the maximum potency of vitamin C permitted in this category would be approximately 60 mg. Higher potencies, such as 250, 500, and 1,000 mg., routinely taken by thousands of Americans, would be reclassified, and if found to have higher health risks would be assigned to Category 3. Amino acids would be assigned to Category 2 and be available by prescription only. Other regulated nutrients and supplements, including many herbs, vitamins, and minerals, found by the FDA to have higher health risks, would be assigned to Category 3 and be available by prescription only. Supplements once readily available over the counter and touted for dramatic health benefits, such as bioflavonoids, rutin, PABA, selenium, inositol, and chromiun, as well as many herbs such as chamomile, would be placed in Category 3 and regulated.

The Task Force's proposal leaked to the public and led to a vigorous outcry. Advocates of nutritional supplements considered it radical, as did many in the medical community. They pointed out that lowering of recommended allowances and restrictions on access to vitamins, minerals, and other supplements came at a time of growing evidence that megadoses of vitamins can help prevent disease. Many in the medical community, alarmed at the megadoses of nutrients and little-understood pharmaceuticals taken by people in the dietary-supplement movement, supported the FDA's proposal to regulate health claims for nutrient supplement doses "not ordinarily consumable." On the other hand, the AMA argued against abandoning the traditional RDA in favor of the lower-dose RDI for minerals and vitamins.

VITAMINS SAFER THAN DRUGS

Only one fatality due to poisonings by vitamin supplements in the United States was reported between 1983 and 1990, according to data from the American Association of Poison Control Centers, and even it was later discovered to be a reporting error. By contrast, in that same period, there were 2,556 fatalities from all major categories of prescription and nonprescription pharmaceutical drugs (with illegal drugs like heroin and cocaine excepted). In fact, the number of deaths zoomed up from 62 in 1983 to 487 in 1990, an increase of almost 700 percent. Thus the statistics suggest that vitamin supplements appear to be approximately 2,500 times safer than drugs. And there may be an even greater safety factor for vitamins, since the statistical trend suggests an increase in pharmaceutical poisonings each year, resulting in a growing disparity between the relative safety of vitamins and the danger of drugs.

Donald C. Loomis
"Which Is Safer: Drugs or Vitamins?"
Townsend Letter for Doctors

Nutritional-supplement enthusiasts pointed to research showing benefits from high doses of many vitamins, especially vitamin C and beta-carotene. Advocates of nutritional supplements charged that NLEA gave the FDA a green light to impose restrictive regulations that prohibited useful health information on labels. They asserted that the regulations violated civil rights by depriving people of the right to get health information and to make up their own minds about personal health issues. The FDA was accused of pushing people into mainstream health care, whether they wanted it or not. Rumors abounded about the FDA and pharmaceutical companies conspiring to establish the "medical-industrial complex" at the expense of the public's health to replace the waning military-industrial complex.

In a letter to the *New York Times* in the summer of 1992, FDA Commissioner Kessler argued back that the agency was not proposing to classify vitamins as drugs based on their potency. He said that the NLEA would not affect sale of high-potency vitamins "as long as they do not pose a health hazard or make misleading medical claims." Kessler pointed to the Proxmire Bill and said that the FDA was not "proposing a specific definition for an upper limit of any substance based on the context of the daily diet." In a follow-up telephone interview, Kessler reiterated that the FDA doesn't "want to discourage the legitimate use of vitamins and minerals to supplement the diet, but we have an obligation," he emphasized, "to discourage unsubstantiated and fraudulent claims." The problem, according to Kessler, is not whether a supplement exceeds the newly established RDI, but whether or not it exceeds "safe levels."

THE FDA ENFORCEMENT AMENDMENTS

The FDA and certain members of Congress felt that new regulations had to be accompanied by increased enforcement powers if the regulations were to be effective. In 1991 Congressmen Waxman (D–California) and Dingell (D–Michigan) in the House and Senator Kennedy (D–Massachusetts) proposed the FDA Amendments (HR 3642/S 2135), commonly called the Waxman Amendment. Under the Amendments the FDA would be able to confiscate products, records, and equipment, levy fines on individuals up to $250,000 and on corporations up to

$1 million, and subpœna records, all without court supervision and without a person having been found guilty of any crime. The effect would be to give the FDA tremendous authority to enforce the NLEA regulations without meeting civil-rights safeguards usually required by due process of law. Because infractions would be viewed as posing health hazards to the public rather than as criminal violations of law-enforcement procedures, the FDA could bypass normal judicial review while seizing property, freezing assets, and preventing businesses from operating.

THE FDA MISSION STATEMENT

It is the FDA's job to see that the food we eat is safe and wholesome, the cosmetics we use won't hurt us, the medicines and medical devices we use are safe and effective, and that radiation-emitting products such as microwave ovens won't do us harm. Feed and drugs for pets and farm animals also come under FDA scrutiny. FDA also ensures that all of these products are labeled truthfully with the information that people need to use them properly.

The Waxman Amendment alarmed a lot of people. Grass-roots efforts mobilized. Thousands of letters and faxes were sent to Senators and Congressmen. Petitions were signed in health-food stores and at New Age fairs. Flyers were mailed. People talked about the coming of the "Vitamin Police." Commissioner Kessler noted in a letter to the *New York Times* that the Administration was opposed to many features of the Waxman Amendment, such as the fines.

THE HEALTH FREEDOM ACT

In response to public alarm, Senator Orrin Hatch (R–Utah) proposed the Health Freedom Act of 1992 (S 2835) and Congressman Bill Richardson (D–New Mexico) proposed the Health Choices Freedom Act (HR 5746) in the House. These acts provide that dietary supplements would not be considered a drug solely because of the substance's potency or because the product literature or label provided information concerning the health claims. The Health Freedom Act would repeal the provisions of the NLEA that permit the establishment of procedures and standards for the validation of disease or health claims required for other foods. Under this act manufacturers would be allowed to provide health-related information on the label or in advertising so long as there is a reasonable scientific basis for the claims, and the information is truthful and not misleading. The FDA would still be authorized to regulate products containing any poisonous or deleterious substance. If a claim made on a label or in advertising is false or misleading, the item would be considered a misbranded food, and the FDA would still have authority to take action against the product.

The bill also provides manufacturers and practitioners with re-course as well as making the FDA more accountable. Under this act, if the FDA issues a warning letter asserting that a disease or health claim is false or misleading or that there is insufficient scientific evidence to support the claim, the manufacturer or practitioner can seek direct judicial review of the merits of FDA's assertion. During the review, the manufacturer will be allowed to continue marketing the product in question, unless it presents a danger to the health of the public. Finally, the act would provide specific standards for dietary supplements.

A fact little known to the public was that before becoming FDA commissioner, Kessler had been a consultant on FDA-related issues to Senator Orrin Hatch, chairman of the Senate Labor and Human Relations committee. Although Kessler did not directly endorse the Hatch Act, he told the *New York Times* in his letter that the new regulations under the NLEA would permit claims to be made on either food or dietary supplements when those claims were supported by "significant scientific consensus." Without such consensus, claims would not be allowed. In fact, the FDA already had the authority to take products off the market if false or misleading claims were made. Under the new labeling act, according to Kessler, manufacturers would be permitted to make health claims if the FDA found the claims were substantiated.

THE FDA VERSUS THE USDA

The NLEA affected all foods, including meats, produce, and dairy products, not just dietary supplements. It was the United States Department of Agriculture's (USDA) responsibility to develop regulations under NLEA for meat and poultry products, and the FDA's responsibility to develop the NLEA for foods, including those found in grocery stores and dietary supplements, as well as for drugs and medical devices. For example, terms like "lite" and "reduced calories" on items found in supermarkets would be strictly defined, serving sizes would be standardized, and complete nutritional information on labels would be mandatory. The dietary-supplement industry was really only a small portion of the target of the labeling reforms.

The thrust of the NLEA was to change the supermarket from a "Tower of Babel," as Louis W. Sullivan, secretary of Health and Human Services called it, to an assembly of clear and coordinated language on product labels. The two agencies were expected to work hand-in-hand in developing the guidelines for what would be required or prohibited on labels. And the two agencies were to create a plan for informing the public about the new label formats. The product of this joint venture was to be in the form of final regulations in November 1992, with manufacturers adhering to the new labels by summer of 1993.

Unfortunately, in the process basic philosophical differences between the two agencies emerged, and they were quickly at loggerheads. Each agency had a different vision of the ideal food label. The FDA favored labels that educate consumers and actively promote a healthful diet. Commissioner Kessler was quoted in *Newsweek* as saying, "The new label is an unusual opportunity to help millions of Americans make more informed, healthier food choices." The USDA and the food industry disagreed. They wanted labels that informed but didn't preach, as they viewed it.

The debate centered on the format and how the nutritional information was to be presented. Interests were polarized, with the FDA and health professionals on one side of the issue, and the USDA and food industry on the other. The FDA's vision was of labels that help people

Nutrition Facts

Serving Size 1/2 cup (114g)

Servings Per Container 4

Amount Per Serving

Calories 260 Calories from Fat 120

% Daily Value*

Total Fat 13g	**20%**
Saturated Fat 5g	**25%**
Cholesterol 30mg	**10%**
Sodium 660mg	**28%**
Total Carbohydrate 31mg	**11%**
Dietary Fiber 0g	**0%**
Sugars 5g	
Protein 5g	

Vitamin A 4% • Vitamin C 2% • Calcium 15% • Iron 4%

*Percents (%) of a Daily Value are based on a 2,000 calorie diet. Your Daily Values may vary higher or lower depending on your calorie needs:

Nutrient		2,000 Calories	2,500 Calories
Total Fat	Less than	65g	80g
Sat Fat	Less than	20g	25g
Cholesterol	Less than	300mg	300mg
Sodium	Less than	2,400mg	2,400mg
Total Carbohydrate		300g	375g
Fiber		25g	30g

1g Fat = 9 calories

1g Carbohydrates = 4 calories

1g Protein = 4 calories

The New Food Label hammered out in a compromise between the FDA and the USDA. It gives consumers information in both absolute terms, like Fat = 13g, and relative terms, like Fat = 20% of Daily Value.

put together a daily diet. Old labels gave such information as the amount of fat in a food. A consumer could compare it with other products to decide which had more or less fat. This information did not help the consumer decide if he or she needed more fat or had fulfilled dietary requirements after eating the product. What the FDA wanted was labels that do just that. They wanted information presented as percentages of the daily dietary requirements in addition to absolute terms. For example, the label would state the amount of fat in a serving and the percentage that it supplies in a diet of 2,000 calories per day. When things are presented in relative terms, which a percentage does, people can make judgments.

The USDA did not like this plan at all. It was called a "grading system" by critics. The USDA said that the percentage format implies that certain foods should be avoided. How meats, which are high in fat, would be labeled was a major stumbling block. People in the meat industry worried that labels with percentages would deter people from eating meat.

The USDA made two counterproposals. The first recommended simply adding a footnote to the old-style label that sums up the U.S. Dietary Guidelines, for example, "Eat a variety of foods and choose foods low in fat." The second proposed that the absolute amount of a nutrient be listed, followed by a range of recommended amounts depending on calorie intake.

At the heart of the controversy was a disagreement about nutritional education. The USDA and the food industry took the position that there are no good foods or bad foods. In their view, all foods can be part of a healthful diet. The FDA, on the other hand, believed that some foods are healthier than others. They wanted the labels to be a tool in educating consumers and helping them to make good dietary decisions. The USDA and their allies didn't agree with that.

November 8, 1992, the deadline for releasing the new guidelines, came and went without resolution of the dispute. Kessler of the FDA threatened that an earlier, more restrictive, proposal would go into law. Finally, the FDA and the USDA took the issue to President Bush, who cut through the Gordian knot with a swift decision a month before leaving office.

Processed foods will show calories, total fat, saturated fat, cholesterol, sodium, carbohydrates, and protein and will be put in the context of a daily diet of 2,000 calories and 65 grams of fat. As a compromise to satisfy Agriculture Secretary Madigam, who had opposed the 2,000-calorie diet, the new labels will also include a 2,500-calorie diet. Each nutrient must be presented as a percentage of a total daily diet. For example, for macaroni and cheese containing 13 grams of fat, the label must also specify that this is 20 percent of the total fat that someone on a 2,000-calorie diet should have for one day. Designations like "low-fat," "high-fiber," and "light" can no longer be used loosely. They must be based on federal definitions. Additionally, serving sizes must be uniform.

Raw meat and poultry are exempt, but products containing meat, such as bologna, must carry the new-style label. Also exempt are restaurant menus—despite Rep. Henry Waxman's (D–California) disapproval.

Health and Human Services Secretary Louis Sullivan estimated that the process of changing hundreds of thousands of labels would cost the food industry about $2 billion.

BREAKING THE DRUG-APPROVAL LOGJAM

The FDA's drug-approval process has traditionally frustrated pharmaceutical companies trying to introduce new products. It can take ten to twelve years with astronomical cost. AIDS sufferers and families of Alzheimer's patients have sharply criticized the slowness of approval, charging that people are dying while the FDA protects them from possible hazards of drugs that might save their lives. In 1992, a creative way through the logjam was proposed that met with widespread support.

The pharmaceutical companies would pay a variety of fees to the FDA for drug approval. The fees would be used to hire six hundred examiners to speed up the review process. The increased staffing would reduce the average time for processing a new drug application from twenty months to twelve, and cut the review time for critically important lifesaving drugs from one year to six months.

It is estimated that pharmaceutical companies lose tens of millions of dollars each month, according to the FDA, as a result of delays in the approval process. Because the government is almost certainly not going to allocate funds to hire the staff needed to speed up the process, the manufacturers elected to pay the bill themselves in the form of fees. Simultaneously, under the new fee procedure continued vigilance of federal safety reviews is ensured.

As the Amendments worked their way through the political hoops in the House and Senate, there came a time when the policies being enforced were not in writing and not actually ratified. Being mandated by Congress under the NLEA, the FDA was compelled to act to protect the public even though the guidelines for the status of drugs, nutrients, herbs, foods, and supplements were in preparation but not fully approved. Likewise, the increased enforcement powers were promised but not confirmed. There was a lot of ambiguity and confusion about what could be said about a substance's health effects, what treatments doctors could prescribe, and what products, including drugs, could be sold. Nonetheless, the FDA put its wheels in motion and hired one hundred special agents to be trained at Quantico, an FBI school for criminal investigation.

The FDA began enforcement actions against high-profile nutritional-supplement manufacturers and practitioners. Raids began with FDA agents, accompanied by local law-enforcement officers, appearing in force, in "drug war" fashion, kicking in doors with guns drawn. Products and equipment were seized, and criminal and civil actions resulted in high legal-defense costs for the people and businesses involved. Often charges were never filed; in other cases the prosecutions were later dropped or defendants won.

Enforcement tactics, such as asset seizures, armed raids, extensive searches, and confiscation of products and records, were the same as those employed by drug-enforcement agencies to carry out the "war on drugs." What was especially frightening was the FDA's ability to close businesses, and take money and property, without having to comply with the legal requirements of the criminal-justice system, such as having to go before a judge prior to acting, reading Miranda Rights to suspects, or allowing them to call attorneys. The "War on Vitamins" was launched.

ILLEGAL PRODUCTS SUBJECT TO SEIZURE

Any product, regardless of its composition, that is clearly associated with smart drug claims—including nutrients and approved or unapproved prescription drugs—is illegal and subject to seizure or other actions by the FDA. Legitimate drugs that affect mental conditions and functions, including those related to aging and memory, must be approved by the FDA before they can be marketed. At this time, no drugs or other products have been approved by the FDA to improve memory or intelligence.

FDA Talk Paper

THE WAR ON VITAMINS

A posse of eleven FDA agents, five U.S. marshals, and four armed Oregon-state police raided Highland Laboratories, a small nutrition company in Mt. Angel, Oregon, in October 1990. Their search warrant specified nine products, but fourteen products were seized, along with labels, artwork, and printing plates for nearly two hundred products. The president, Ken Scott, was prevented from entering the building, and the staff was detained for four hours. Scott's records for nonrelated business activities were also seized because he was providing literature about Highland's nutritional products to clients requesting the information. More than a year later Scott's records were still being held, even though no criminal charges had been filed against him.

A couple of months after the Highland Labs' raid, on January 9, 1991, the FDA said that Life Extension International in Phoenix was selling "misbranded" products. They raided and confiscated forty-two nutritional supplements—all of them considered legal under current rulings. With the help of seven lawyers and a private investigator working twelve days, Life Extension International persuaded the court to lift the injunction and restraining order on selling its products, and survived.

ENTREPRENEURIAL VITAMIN CHEMISTS

A police sergeant and twelve FDA agents, some armed with guns, appeared in May 1991 at the San Leandro, California, office of Stephen Levine, a biochemist trained at UC Berkeley and author of *Antioxidant Adaptation: Its Role in Free Radical Pathology*. They claimed that his company, Nutricology, Inc., was selling illegal drugs and engaging in mail and wire fraud. They searched his office, warehouse, and computer records looking for the evidence for two days. Nutricology assets were frozen, and sales were halted for two weeks.

Nutricology was able to get back into business when Judge D. Lowell Jensen of the U.S. District Court for the Northern District of California overturned the government's preliminary injunction and temporary restraining order. In his decision he stated that there was insufficient evidence for serious, irreparable harm resulting from allowing Nutricology to continue to sell its products. He said that issuing a permanent injunction would threaten to destroy the company, since the targeted products represented about 80 percent of Nutricology's business. Jensen pointed out that the FDA had been fighting the company for nine years, which clearly indicated that there was no "new and unexpected, much less irreparable, harm" from the company continuing to market its products, and noted that the government was "unable to show even a single instance where a consumer was injured" as a result of any of the products.

While Nutricology continued in business, the government continued trying to get yet another injunction, the fourth, against it. Nutricology has been fighting on, spending more than $300,000 in legal-defense fees in the year of the raid.

Dr. Robert Koch is another biochemist targeted by the FDA. He developed a series of products called Vitacel that are similar to

Gerovital used by Dr. Ana Aslan in the 1950s in her famous Romanian youth clinic. Because of earlier problems, Koch had stopped producing Vitacel in the U.S. It was available only from Nutritional Engineering, Ltd. (NEL), in the Cayman Islands in the British West Indies. Mail orders were received in Seattle and forwarded to NEL in Grand Cayman until May 1991, when about a dozen FDA and U.S. Postal Service agents, accompanied by armed police, entered the agency, seized all mail directed to NEL, and seized NEL's Oregon bank account. Simultaneously, in South Jordan, Utah, FDA agents, police, and federal marshals charged into Koch's home. They detained his daughter and granddaughter for twelve hours while they searched. They seized his computer and research records, which represented his life's work, along with data discs, computer software, and personal and business records. Additionally, Koch said they seized his personal bank account, began monitoring his mail, tapped his phones, and followed him and his family members. The FDA claimed that Koch was engaged in mail fraud and money laundering.

Mail-fraud charges were eventually dropped, and the FDA threatened but never charged Koch with a crime. Like Levine and Nutricology, Koch and NEL continued in business.

HEALTH GURUS

In Kent, Washington, just outside of Seattle, on the morning of May 6, 1992, as Dr. Jonathan Wright was about to open for the day the Tahoma Clinic, an alternative health center, there was a pounding at the door. Before his staff could answer it, more than a dozen FDA agents and King County sheriffs burst through the door, some wearing flak vests, with guns drawn, crying out for everyone to freeze. One pointed a gun at the receptionist, telling her to "Get your hands up where I can see them," while another yanked out the telephone lines when a staffer tried to make a call. As patients came in, upset employees, one crying and another who was later treated for heart palpitations, looked on as agents searched the office and pored through the files. They seized various vitamin and nutrient supplements, along with medical and business equipment, and business and patient records. That same morning they

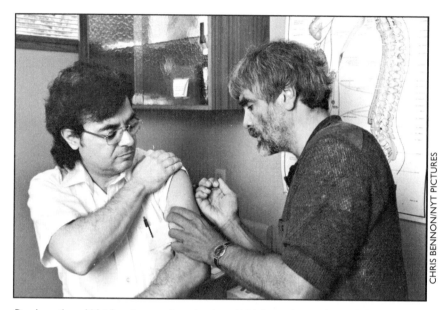

Dr. Jonathan Wright gives a vitamin shot. Wright is the author of Guide to Healing and is on the board of directors of the Seattle-based John Bastyr College of Naturopathic Medicine and of the National Health Federation.

also raided a nearby pharmacy, For Your Health Pharmacy, which filled prescriptions and dispensed other nutrient products for Wright and other doctors.

Although Wright was not formally charged with any crime, the FDA alleged that he was smuggling drugs into the U.S. and manufacturing drugs without a license. Wright disagreed. He said the pharmacy and laboratory supplying the clinic were using natural vitamins, minerals, and herbs obtained through commercial suppliers and mixing special formulations for doctors by prescription. Wright protested that it was ridiculous for the FDA to accuse him of producing drugs and to raid his clinic as if it were a "crack house."

The "drug" that the FDA said Wright was smuggling was a preservative-free injectable B_{12} legally used in Germany, but not approved for use in the U.S. Wright, who was educated at Harvard and the University of Michigan Medical School, said he was treating people with allergies who could not tolerate the preservatives in the B_{12} available in the U.S.

The FDA said it was concerned with the sterility of the product, especially since it was being injected.

PRACTICING MEDICINE WITH ONE HAND TIED
One of my greatest frustrations in nutritional-biochemical practice is knowing that there are many serious illnesses that could be helped or even prevented, right now, by nutritional, biochemical, and other holistic means. But it isn't being done. I'm forced to practice medicine with one hand tied behind my back.

Dr. Jonathan Wright

Additionally, the FDA accused Wright of using a machine called the "Interro" for diagnosis. The machine, which has not been approved for therapeutic use in the U.S., uses electronic sensors attached to a finger to measure galvanic skin response as a test for food allergies. The machine, which has been approved for research only, was used at the Tahoma Clinic on an FDA undercover agent who had gained the treatment by posing as a patient. Wright insisted that using the device was better than "injecting people to see if they swell up," which is the medically approved method of testing for allergies.

Wright contended that the FDA raid was in retaliation for his ongoing lawsuit against the FDA. He sued the FDA for the return of his supply of L-tryptophan used as a dietary supplement. His supply was seized when the FDA recalled all L-tryptophan after a series of mysterious illnesses were linked to the food supplement. Because the Centers for Disease Control later discovered that the illnesses were caused by a contaminant in a particular line of L-tryptophan products, Wright asserted that the FDA had no cause to seize and hold his L-tryptophan supply, which was uncontaminated. Wright believed the raid was motivated by this continuing lawsuit, as well as his non-traditional practices, with the objective of putting him out of business. The FDA claimed it didn't care about Wright's practicing alternative therapies, only whether or not his therapies were hazardous to health.

Wright had also been having problems with the IRS, which had decided that tax shelters he had invested in in the 1970s were not allowed, and had filed $400,000 in tax liens against him. Wright asserted that his problems with the IRS were connected with his problems with the FDA. When he held a news conference a few days after the raid to protest the FDA's tactics, Wright's attorney recognized two IRS officers in the audience. Wright's supporters cried foul, but the FDA said it wasn't working in conjunction with the IRS.

FDA Commissioner Kessler challenged the widely publicized accounts of the raid at the Tahoma Clinic, which reported that armed agents had burst into the clinic. He said, "No FDA employees were armed, although one local sheriff drew his gun as a precautionary measure." The agents had a search warrant. Kessler said the warrant was necessary because the clinic officials had refused earlier requests to inspect it. Clinic officials pointed out that they were merely exercising their Constitutional rights. In an interview to the *New York Times*, Kessler said, "We were more concerned about the sterility and safety of the products being used by Dr. Jonathan Wright, founder of the clinic, than in his practice of medicine."

THE 1960S REVISITED

The targeting of a vitamin guru like Wright to make an example of him is a familiar drug-enforcement approach. For example, Timothy Leary, the 1960s psychedelic guru, was targeted by drug-enforcement officials, even before LSD was made illegal. He was sentenced to thirty years, after the remains from a marijuana cigarette were found in his car's ashtray during a search.

Curiously, the FDA's war on vitamins came at a time when the war on drugs was being denounced by many as a failure, and debates raged about legalizing drugs in order to halt the police-state-type enforcement tactics. In the early 1990s increasing numbers of people were questioning the loss of civil rights to the cause of the war on drugs. Even some conservative figures, including well-known right-wing journalist and pundit William F. Buckley, Jr., and former Secretary of State George

Schultz came out in favor of drug legalization. Within this context, the war on vitamins seemed to be repeating history.

WILL VITAMINS BE DECLARED ILLICIT?

Before the psychedelic movement of the middle and late 1960s, many psychoactive agents were readily obtainable from legitimate chemical companies. Unlike marijuana, cocaine, and other "street drugs" of minority cultures, exotic substances such as ibogaine, psilocybin, and dimethyltryptamine had not, in the eyes of the authorities, presented any social problem. Virtually no one had even heard of them. In October 1970, under Title 21 of the United States Code, many of these "unheard-of" substances became illicit.

Mind drugs, though, are not the only materials that the federal government has declared war on. The FDA has been trying for years to control sales of ordinary vitamins, and to limit the allowable dosages of pills to almost useless amounts. Most of their attempts in this direction have been defeated so far. Nevertheless, they had some victories.

John Mann
Secrets of Life Extension

OTHER AREAS OF INCREASED ENFORCEMENT

The FDA stepped up enforcement of laws already on the books, interpreting them more strictly to permit it to act. Many of these actions affected products used for other than brain-boosting efforts, but the writing on the wall was clear that the FDA was taking a stronger role in regulating everything. For example, in the Summer of 1992, the FDA went after a northern California winery because it claimed on its label that, according to a French study, a glass of wine a day helped reduce heart attacks. The wine industry rallied around and protested that the FDA was interfering with their free speech. Around the same time the

FDA forced Kraft Foods to remove a salad dressing from the market because its name, "Heart Lite," implied that its low-cholesterol content would help reduce heart disease. The FDA did not, however, employ the Gestapo-like enforcement tactics used during the raids against Wright, Nutricology, and others in the nutrient-supplement business.

TIGHTENING UP POLICIES ON MAIL IMPORTATIONS OF DRUGS

At the same time, the FDA began to tighten up the personal exemption allowing individuals to get unapproved products from foreign sources where they are legal. In response to AIDS activists, there was a policy of allowing people to acquire drugs for treatment of serious and life-threatening conditions like AIDS and Alzheimer's from other countries where they are readily available over the counter or through clinics, or sold mail order by off-shore suppliers. Although there never was a guarantee that these drugs and nutrients would be permitted across the border, a 1988 FDA policy directive gave enforcers the discretion to examine the background, risk, and purpose of these products. The policy was to not detain articles without substantial reasons, such as suspicions that the drugs or nutrients might be for commercial use, or when the department had issued an Import Alert about a specific product. Products could be imported without sampling or detention if intended for personal use, in no more than a three-month supply. The intended use of the substance was supposed to be identified, and the name and address of a doctor licensed in the U.S. treating the importer was to be included. Enforcement of these rules was lax.

With the extraordinary press coverage of Dean and Morgenthaler's book *Smart Drugs & Nutrients* came more scrutiny. About the book FDA Consumer Affairs Officer Mary-Margaret Richardson stated, "The philosophy behind this book really stinks." Morgenthaler thumbed his nose at the FDA. During interviews on national prime-time television shows like *Nightline,* he held up boxes of imported drugs like hydergine and piracetam, and described their wondrous effects on memory and cognition. Morgenthaler was very vocal in his disdain for the FDA's regulations. He readily encouraged interested people to investigate the

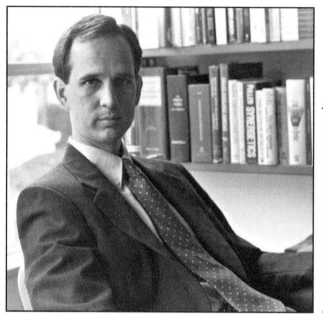

John Morgenthaler, author of Smart Drugs & Nutrients *(with Ward Dean) and* Stop The FDA *(with Steven Fowkes), is a proponent of health freedom who has spoken out against FDA actions.*

buyer's clubs, and supplied addresses in the book.

Early in 1992, the FDA began to tighten up the enforcement of this exception, making it more difficult for people to import foreign prod-ucts, especially pharmaceuticals, for personal use. People who had previously obtained smart drugs from foreign labs received notices from the FDA informing them that they could no longer import them. Gary Dykstra, the FDA's deputy associate commissioner for Regulatory Affairs, said that packages coming from known suppliers of smart drugs and other pharmaceuticals would be subject to more scrutiny. He indicated that certain drugs such as THA for Alzheimer's patients would be allowed if accompanied by a doctor's prescription and a description of the condition being treated.

Morgenthaler criticized the FDA, saying that the FDA was "woe-fully behind the times" in approving state-of-the-art smart drugs and other medically proven treatments. He described the FDA's position as being oriented toward treatment of disease only, rather than toward maintenance or improvement of health. He said that the real issue is whether or not people can have the freedom to make personal choices about what they can put into their bodies. In an interview with *High Times Magazine* in September 1992, Morgenthaler advised overseas pharmaceutical suppliers to "disappear and pop up with a new name and address. The FDA is slow, clumsy, and inflexible. They take about a year to ban a company, and by that time the company can pop up again with a new identity."

The nutritional industry has been largely unregulated, and the illnesses and deaths from tryptophan provided a trigger to increase the FDA regulation of this multibillion-dollar industry. According to Health Foods Business, a trade organization, the vitamin and nutrition industry has $1.46 billion in sales through health-food stores alone. The market for nutrients more than doubled in the 1980s, becoming a major force in over-the-counter pharmaceuticals and selling billions more through mail order and multilevel marketing channels.

The FDA's concern is the potential for abuse in a booming, unregulated industry. There have been some questionable practices, such as promising unsubstantiated cures, ads misrepresenting products, improper endorsements, and inappropriate quotes of research results. Sick people can be exploited by unscrupulous claims that discredit the industry.

Critics say the FDA's "drug war" tactics do not adequately distinguish between people responsibly selling and promoting legitimate products and the exploiters making false claims. Big medical institutions and pharmaceutical companies are eyeing the growing popularity of the nutritional approaches to health and the billions of dollars to be made. Some fear that these companies are using their influence with the FDA to make sure that this money goes into their own coffers, not to small new firms or independent contractors.

7

NOOTROPICS

Smart pharmaceuticals run the gamut from memory and learning enhancers to drugs used to slow down aging, to counteract certain disease conditions that interfere with intelligence, or to generally stimulate the central nervous systems. Classifying smart pharmaceuticals into different categories is not straightforward, since there is overlap in uses and in how they act on the brain, nervous system, and body to achieve their purposes. Nootropics are pharmaceuticals that can enhance learning and memory. A drug designed to slow down aging could, in the process, improve memory and learning, but not be classified as a nootropic which are specifically intended to act on the brain. Because of this confusion, it is helpful to get an overview of the growing number of smart drugs that are out there.

Nootropics are pharmaceuticals that improve learning, memory, and recall without other effects on the central nervous system. The term *nootropic* comes from Greek roots meaning "acting on the mind." According to Dean and Morgenthaler, nootropics were first described in 1972 by C. E. Giurgia in a French pharmacological journal.

Nootropics work by acting on the chemicals that carry impulses or messages between brain cells. They promote production of the all-important neurotransmitters, such as acetylcholine, which facilitates the transmission of messages from one neuron to another in the brain.

Nootropics can prevent the kind of mental deterioration that comes with aging and is caused by declining production of neurotransmitters.

Be cautioned about overdoses. The fact that nootropics stimulate neurological transmittal doesn't mean that the more you take, the faster the transmittal and the better you can think. As with many drugs, there is an optimum point at which the effects peak and then drop off. There is some evidence that you can overdose if you take too much. Should you take a nootropic, it's important to find out the optimum dosage to get the most benefit. One nootropic may interact with other pharmaceuticals and over-the-counter medications as well as herbs and nutrients. Combinations may reduce the amount of the nootropic or other substances required for gaining the optimum desired effects.

DIAGNOSIS IS FOR PROFESSIONALS

CAUTION: **Before you assume that any declining mental functions are really due to your age, be sure to consult with your doctor. Increasing forgetfulness, being "too tired" to learn something new, and other symptoms may in fact be due to other conditions such as anemia and diabetes mellitus. If you practice "self-diagnosis," you might be wrong and neglect an important medical disorder. Diagnosis is definitely for professionals.**

Durk Pearson and Sandy Shaw
Life Extension

Whether you should use smart drugs and, if so, which and how much, is not a question we can answer for the reader. Each person's body and chemistry are different, and the drugs have not been through the complete testing required by the FDA. The wisest course is to consult a knowledgeable physician before taking any drug, and certainly cognitive-enhancement programs should be carried out under the direction of a knowledgeable physician. A list of such physicians can be found in the Appendix. Dean and Morgenthaler, authors of *Smart Drugs & Nutrients*, also maintain a list of physicians who have expertise

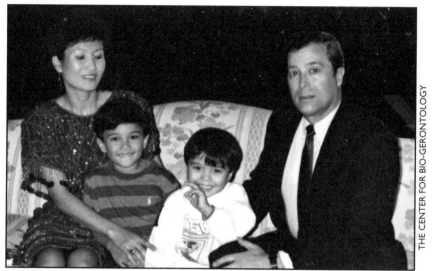

Pioneering gerontological researcher, Ward Dean, M.D. *(shown with his family) is author of* Biological Aging Measurement, Smart Drugs & Nutrients *(with John Morgenthaler), and* The Neuroendocrine Theory of Aging and Degenerative Disease *(with Vladimir Dilman).*

in this area. Our purpose here is merely to provide an overview of smart pharmaceuticals, of their potential benefits and hazards, and of how some people have used them.

PYRROLIDONE

Nootropics are categorized by chemical composition and the different ways they act to speed up mental processing. One class of nootropics is derived from pyrrolidone, a substance that affects the parts of the nervous system that use acetylcholine as a neurotransmitter, and are sometimes referred to as the *cholinergic system.* Acetylcholine controls sensory signals and muscle contraction, and plays an important role in memory and learning. The drugs in this class include piracetam and its analogs oxiracetam, pramiracetam, and aniracetam. Analogs are molecules with similar molecular structure.

Piracetam. Piracetam, also called nootropil, is the most commonly taken nootropic. It helps boost intelligence without being toxic or addictive. Being the first nootropic drug to be developed, it gave rise to this whole new category of drugs. Piracetam is very similar in chemical structure to the amino acid pyroglutamate, present in meat, vegetables, fruits, and dairy products.

It is in the cerebral cortex that thought and reasoning are believed to occur. Piracetam stimulates the cerebral cortex and increases the rate of metabolism and energy level of brain cells. It does not have the side effects associated with other stimulants. The primary clinical use is to protect the brain from damage caused by hypoxia, which is oxygen starvation, and to help recover from it. Brain cells can be starved for oxygen by drinking too much alcohol, for example. Another clinical use is stemming memory loss caused by physical injury and chemical poisoning.

Piracetam seems to help step up the flow of messages between the two hemispheres or halves of the brain, which is sometimes called the *interhemispheric flow of information.* In fact, psychopharmacologist Dr. Dimond said the brains of subjects who used piracetam seemed "superconnected," which he attributed to an increased exchange between hemispheres.

Dean and Morgenthaler speculate that the increased communication between right and left brains is associated with flashes of creativity. If their hypothesis is correct, then piracetam not only improves memory and ability to learn, but has the potential to enhance creativity as well.

Improved transfer between brain hemispheres occurs because piracetam stimulates the cerebral cortex to increase production of a compound called adenosine triphosphate (ATP) in the brain cells. The buildup and breakdown of ATP produces energy in the cells. The amount of ATP that is available to be turned into energy declines with aging. It is believed that piracetam reverses this process by increasing the activity of the enzyme that produces ATP.

According to Dean and Morgenthaler, piracetam may actually have a regenerative effect on the nervous system. They point to a study by Pitch, who found that piracetam improves brain functioning in mice by increasing the number of cholinergic receptors in the brain.

Piracetam may improve learning by increasing the brain's ability to synthesize new proteins. According to Pelton, author of *Mind Foods and*

Smart Pills, information or learning is encoded into the new proteins. Researchers believe piracetam manufactures new proteins by stimulating certain structures within the cells called polyribosomes. The specific chain of events is complicated and beyond the scope of this book, but the upshot of the research is that piracetam is a powerful nootropic that seems to contribute to improved memory and learning through several different types of chemical changes that it triggers in the brain.

PIRACETAM MAY HELP MARIJUANA USERS
While there seem to be no studies specifically related to marijuana, many agents which impair learning such as physical injury, oxygen deprivation, and barbiturates have been shown to be mediated by piracetam. There are good reasons to believe that marijuana memory impairment would also show mediation, but marijuana research is not sufficiently respectable these days to warrant "serious" effort. This is regrettable. Although there are anecdotal reports in the "popular" literature which suggests that piracetam mediates marijuana memory impairment, this is utterly unscientific and should not be used as a reason for taking piracetam.

Nootropic News

Researchers studying performance have gotten positive results in tests on both animals and humans using piracetam. Animals have been found to learn faster and better when given piracetam. One group of rats consuming piracetam were better able to avoid a small shock. Studies with human volunteers by Dimond and Browers and by Mindus found performance improvements in students, young and healthy volunteers, and middle-aged subjects suffering some memory loss, all of whom showed significant improvements in memory and mental performance.

Research indicates that piracetam has a synergistic effect, such as helping the individual remember things better, when taken with DMAE, centrophenoxine, choline, Deaner, lecithin, or hydergine. Reports show it works three to four times better when acetylcholine-enhancing nutrients or drugs are used.

Piracetam is especially effective in enhancing memory when used with choline. Dr. Pelton asserts that combining the nutrient choline and the drug piracetam "may be the most potent memory-enhancing therapy yet discovered." Studies suggest that when taken in combination, the two substances are much more effective both in improving memory and in preventing the mental decline that comes with aging than when either substance is used by itself.

Dr. Raymond Bartus showed this remarkable effect in a study on rats. A subject rat was shocked, then after twenty-four hours returned to the same dark chamber where it was shocked again. Whereas older rats are worse at remembering the shock than younger rats, Bartus found that when given choline plus piracetam the rats, both young and old, were significantly better at remembering and so waited longer to enter the chamber and get shocked. Impressed by these findings with rats, Ferris and some associates at NYU's psychiatry department tried a similar experiment on humans suffering from Alzheimer's disease. They found a tremendous increase in memory as shown by their scores on a verbal memory test when the two substances were used together. Performance on one test went up *70 percent* in subjects taking piracetam plus choline.

Researchers now believe that choline is an important substance to use with any of the nootropic drugs. The theory is that nootropics stimulate the cholinergic neurons, which are the cells in the brain that produce the neurotransmitter acetylcholine, which promotes thought and memory. When this happens, the level of choline in the cell is reduced. The faster the neuron fires and/or the lower the amount of choline in the cells, the more the choline is depleted. When the supply gets too low, the cholinergic neuron will break down its own membrane to obtain the choline it needs to make more acetylcholine. Consuming its own membrane is known as *autocannibalism* and will eventually kill the cell if it continues. Taking choline, however, increases the choline

level, and the cells continue to make the necessary acetylcholine
without consuming their own membrane.

SMART DRUGS INSTEAD OF COFFEE

**I've come to use hydergine and piracetam much in the way
that I used to use coffee, but without any of the nasty side
effects that I experienced from caffeine. Both increase my
mental clarity, alertness, improve my concentration, enhance my memory, sharpen my verbal acuity, and can even
be used synergistically for a unique effect unlike either on
their own. But it's hydergine, in particular, that acts as a
mild antidepressant. Piracetam has the added feature of
increasing my auditory sensitivity, much in the way that
marijuana does, without the high, and allows me to experience heightened attentiveness to detail when listening to
music.**

Dave Brown
High Times Magazine

In any case, the research indicates that either by itself or with
choline, piracetam is one of the most effective nootropic drugs in its
impact on memory and learning. People generally take 800 to 1,600 mg.
of piracetam a day. They often begin with a higher dose, of 1,200 to 2,400
mg., taken in the early part of the day for the first two days, and then
lower the dose thereafter. It is not toxic and has no contraindications.
However, Dean and Morgenthaler do report that it can sometime
increase the effects of amphetamines, psychotropics, and hydergine.
Piracetam is most easily obtained over the counter in Mexico and in
various European countries. Sometimes it can be obtained through the
mail from an off-shore pharmacy.

Oxiracetam. Chemically, oxiracetam is similar to piracetam,
though stronger in effect. It is one of the more commonly used smart

drugs, and known by a number of names, including CT-848, hydroxypiracetam, ISF-2522, Neuractiv, and Neuromet.

Oxiracetam has had the most widespread use in Italy, where it was developed in 1988 by ICF, an Italian drug company. By the early 1990s, its use was spreading to other European countries, as well as Japan. Meanwhile, in the U.S., use has not been approved by the FDA. SmithKline Beckman Corporation is trying to get the drug approved for treating Alzheimer's disease.

Oxiracetam has been tested on both mice and people in Europe, Japan, and the U.S. One of the mice tests in Japan showed that it takes less oxiracetam than piracetam to improve learning (only about a third as much). In another study, in Italy, the newborn mice of mothers given oxiracetam turned out to be more curious when they were born, and remembered more in memory tests than did the offspring of mothers who didn't get such a boost.

The tests on humans show similar favorable results. When elderly subjects with dementia, a disease of aging, were tested, researchers found the effects of oxiracetam were greater than those of piracetam in improving ability to remember things. These results have been replicated a number of times.

There has been very little research on normal, healthy people, however. The premise underlying research on animals or special groups of people is that its results can be generalized to the larger population. But to date we don't know if the generalization to healthy people holds. Oxiracetam has been shown to be nontoxic, like other nootropics, as well as safe in dosages that far exceed what the average person takes— 1,200 to 2,400 mg. a day seems to be the usual dose for improvements in cognitive functioning.

Pramiracetam. Pramiracetam, also known as CI-879, is another chemical relative to piracetam, and has a similar effect in improving the operations of the neurotransmitter acetylcholine. Like oxiracetam, pramiracetam appears to be more potent than piracetam. A lower dose can be used to achieve the same effect. A study with Alzheimer's patients revealed that both piracetam and pramiracetam improve intelligence and memory. However, the researchers had to use about fifteen times as much piracetam to get the same effect, leading to the conclusion that pramiracetam is about fifteen times more powerful. Most studies show that pramiracetam is more effective than piracetam in treating Alzheimer's patients. Doses range from 150 to 300 mg.

Although pramiracetam seems to be more potent and effective, it is less common than piracetam. Pramiracetam is newer, less tested, and less available. Parke Davis is working through the maze of FDA approval of pramiracetam to treat Alzheimer's disease. If pramiracetam becomes legally available, it will probably be used not only for Alzheimer's disease but for cognitive enhancement as well.

Aniracetam. Aniracetam, another chemical cousin of piracetam, is also known as Draganon, Ro 13-5057, and Sarpul. It is considered even more powerful, and is used to treat more conditions. Aniracetam has much the same effect as piracetam without problems of toxicity or side effects, according to Dean and Morgenthaler. Its use as a smart drug is less common. The U.S. patent holder, Hoffman-LaRoche, has had problems gaining FDA approval for treating Alzheimer's disease. Hoffman-LaRoche assigned the rights to foreign companies, but so far the drug has not been officially approved in any country. Though it has great potential, aniracetam is primarily used in research, and is not yet widely available as a smart drug.

Pyroglutamate (PCA). Pyroglutamate is another member of the pyrrolidone family, and is also chemically similar to piracetam. Pyroglutamate has many names, such as PCA (2-oxo-pyrrolidon carboxylic acid), alpha-aminoglutaric acid lactam, glutamic acid lactam, glutimic acid, glutiminic acid, pyroGlu, and pyroglutamic acid. Although it may be classified as a drug, pyroglutamate is used in nutrient-type products sold in health stores under various trade names, such as Amino Mass, Mental Edge, and Deep Thought. Doses range from 400 to 1,000 mg. a day. Sometimes pyroglutamate is sold in the form of a growth-hormone stimulant, known as arginine pyroglutamate, which is used to improve cognition and sold under trade names like Adjuvant,

DOSE DETERMINATION

1. Keep good records of the substances you use and your clinical laboratory test results. With records, you can follow the course of your experimental program to find out how you have benefited, to adjust dosages, to add new materials to your experiment, and to avoid further use of materials to which you are sensitive.

2. Before you begin using any new nutrients or drugs, you should have a set of clinical laboratory tests run to establish baselines of body functions.

3. Begin taking the substance at the low end of the expected therapeutic-dose range and work your dose up *slowly*. Notice how you feel as you use a dose for a week to several weeks. Then increase the dose by 50 percent or so at a time. For prescription drugs, do not make any changes without discussing this with your physician.

4. Have clinical laboratory tests taken at intervals, such as once every three to six months, or at the very least once a year.

5. A good way to find your proper dose is to continue increasing the dose *slowly* until you reach an acceptable level of harmless and reversible side effects. Reduce the dosage somewhat when you reach this point, until you do feel comfortable. This is often a good personalized *maximum* dosage.

6. Under times of stress and/or illness, your requirements for many nutrients will be higher.

7. Above all, be patient. Don't try to establish your entire program in one month. Add one new item to your regimen at a time. Change your dosage by one item at a time. Keep your physician informed, and be sure to discuss prescriptions with him or her.

8. To reduce dosages, it is important to *taper off gradually* rather than stop all at once when reducing dosages of water-soluble nutrients.

Durk Pearson and Sandy Shaw
Life Extension

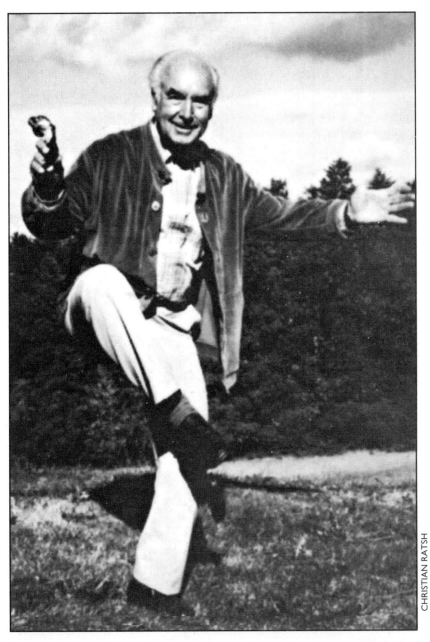

CHRISTIAN RATSH

Sandoz research chemist, Albert Hoffmann, who first extracted hydergine from ergot rye, holds a ling chi mushroom while practicing Tai Chi on his 80th birthday.

Piraglutargine, and Arginine Pidolate. It has been shown to be effective in helping people with alcohol-induced memory deficits.

You might wonder how pyroglutamate gained all this widespread availability, whereas other drugs in the piracetam family are still struggling to gain approval. One reason is that while it is chemically similar to other nootropics, it also is an amino acid, and is found commonly in natural foods, including vegetables, fruits, dairy products, and meats. We regularly eat pyroglutamate in foods. In fact, the brain, the fluid surrounding the brain, and the blood contain this amino acid. Thus, despite its chemical similarities to substances classified as drugs, pyroglutamate is more like a nutrient, although in concentrated form it might become considered a drug. Pyroglutamate passes through the blood-brain barrier into the brain, where it stimulates thinking, memory, and learning.

Various improvements have been found in tests on both rats and people taking pyroglutamate. In one study, people with a loss of memory due to alcohol remembered more when they used pyroglutamate. Elderly people who suffered from dementia were better able to pay attention and recall things when using pyroglutamate. Older people who experienced simple memory decline due to normal aging reported improved memories when taking pyroglutamate. Pyroglutamate has also been found to increase the size of muscles as a growth hormone stimulant. Like most nootropics, pyroglutamate has been found to be nontoxic and safe. With all these benefits, no wonder pyroglutamate is popular, has many names, and is sold in many different forms.

HYDERGINE

The easiest to obtain of the brain-boosting drugs is hydergine. It is made up of a combination of three different ergot alkaloids, derived from a fungus called *Claviceps purpurea* that grows on rye. One of the interesting things about hydergine is that it is chemically similar to LSD, which is also derived from the ergot rye fungus. Both of these alkaloids were discovered by Albert Hoffmann in the 1940s.

NON-SMOKERS ARE SMARTER

Lung diseases like pneumonia, chronic obstructive lung disease, and lung cancer are conditions that reduce the amount of oxygen in the bloodstream. They are all diseases associated with cigarette smoking. Smoking, even without lung disease, reduces the amount of oxygen in the blood, because of gases like carbon monoxide inhaled with the cigarette smoke.

Tobacco cigarettes are the most addictive drug in the world. It is more addictive and harder to "kick" than heroin. Nicotine is one of the strongest stimulants known. Smoking is an efficient method of drug delivery that puts drugs into the brain more directly than intravenous injection.

When cigarettes were first introduced, they were promoted as a healthy way to stimulate mental alertness and relaxation. In fact, nicotine constricts blood vessels and interferes with circulation throughout the body, including the brain. Hence oxygen supply to the brain is reduced, which has a direct negative impact on mental functioning. Chronic smokers suffer brain-cell death from oxygen depletion. Further, free radicals are created with each breath of smoke. Adding to its negatives is that cigarette smoke is one of the richest-known sources of carcinogenic agents, which are carried directly into the brain! Dr. Andrew Weil strongly suggests that anyone who has been a chronic smoker in the last ten years take 25,000 units of beta-carotene a day.

Hydergine is considered by some to be an all-purpose brain booster. It increases mental abilities, prevents brain cells from being damaged by free radicals or by too little oxygen (hypoxia), and reverses brain-cell damage. Hydergine increases learning, memory, and recall in several ways. It speeds up the level of metabolism in the brain cells and increases the amount of blood and oxygen getting to the brain. Hydergine reduces brain damage when oxygen is insufficient, as during a stroke. Hydergine slows down lipofuscin deposits associated with brain-cell aging, and acts as a prophylactic against damage from free radicals.

The only FDA-approved uses of hydergine are senility and cerebrovascular insufficiency, which is caused by poor blood circulation to the brain. Hydergine's effectiveness in reducing symptoms of senility have been well-established. The FDA has approved dosages up to 3 mg. per day only. Dr. Pelton's review of the literature suggested that 3 mg. per day is not enough for most people suffering reduced blood circulation to the brain. A higher dose, of 4.5 to 6 mg. per day, appears to be more effective. In Europe, however, physicians can prescribe higher dosages, up to 9 mg. per day, and can use it preventively with patients who have mild mental deterioration.

Hydergine increases the oxygen supply in the brain, which keeps production of free radicals in check. When oxygen is in short supply because of smoking, cerebral insufficiency, strokes, or heart attacks, free radicals are rapidly produced, resulting in brain-cell damage.

A famous study on cats dramatizes hydergine's remarkable ability to protect brain cells. Two groups of cats, one treated with hydergine and one without, were anesthetized and subjected to reduced oxygen and blood to the brain. Within five minutes, the cats without hydergine had some brain damage; the treated cats did not. After fifteen minutes the nontreated cats were virtually dead from the tremendous and irreversible brain damage they suffered. Here's the astonishing finding. The cats getting hydergine still showed strong brain waves. Even after forty-five minutes of deprivation, the hydergine cats still reacted like normal cats without any brain damage! This study demonstrated that hydergine reduces damage from free radicals, even when the oxygen supply to the brain is dramatically reduced.

In Europe, hydergine is regularly given in hospital emergency rooms to victims of strokes, heart attacks, hemorrhage, drug overdoses, drowning, and electrocution. Because brain damage can occur from emergencies during surgery where oxygen and blood can be cut off, European hospitals routinely administer hydergine pre-surgery as an extra measure of caution. In spite of the volumes of research demonstrating the effectiveness of hydergine in these cases, use with accident victims or as a preventive measure is not approved in the United States by the FDA.

Healthy people can benefit from hydergine use. For example, in one study, young, healthy volunteers taking higher than normal dosages (12 mg. per day) for two weeks showed greater alertness and thinking abilities. Early data from a longitudinal study with about 150 healthy elderly people confirm that when taken regularly, hydergine helps to maintain physical and mental health. Dr. Pelton enthusiastically concludes that hydergine "slows down the aging process." Furthermore, hydergine does not have any serious side effect. When mild side effects such as headaches, dizziness, or nausea do occur, they are due to starting therapy with large dosages rather than gradually working up to a higher dose. Pelton does caution, however, that although hydergine is virtually nontoxic, it should not be used by anyone with psychosis.

Hydergine has been studied extensively, with more than 3,000 research papers published on it to date, making it one of the most widely studied and prescribed drugs. Hydergine was originally produced and distributed by Sandoz Pharmaceuticals, and later by Dorsey Pharmaceuticals, a division of Sandoz. Because the original patent has expired, numerous generic versions are now available in various strengths through prescription. According to FDA guidelines, prescription is permitted for anti-senility only. However, in practice it is often used for improving intelligence and combating aging, and is prescribed for higher doses than those usually approved in the U.S.

Hydergine is available in the U.S. by prescription only. Hydergine may have even better effects when used in conjunction with piracetam; researchers suggest taking smaller doses of both to get the best effect.

VASOPRESSIN

Vasopressin has memory-enhancing effects and is widely known as the prescription drug manufactured by Sandoz Pharmaceutical Company under the trade name Diapid. Vasopressin is a brain hormone produced in the pituitary gland, and acts to imprint new information into the brain's memory centers. Without vasopressin you can't learn or acquire new information. Similarly, it helps in memory retrieval by drawing information into conscious thought.

Earliest research was conducted in the Netherlands in the mid-'60s by Dr. de Wied, who found that vasopressin acts directly on brain cells and the central nervous system to improve the imprinting system by which electric impulses with information became encoded into long-term memories. During this process new proteins are synthesized and deposited into the memory centers of the brain. He demonstrated that animals given vasopressin exhibited improved memory retention, greater ability to learn, some protection against memory loss due to injuries from either chemical or physical causes, and better retrieval of memories lost because of amnesia. When de Wied gave vasopressin to animals suffering congenital deficiencies of the hormone, their severe memory deficiencies were reversed.

Research on humans using vasopressin revealed similar memory-enhancing results. Studies range from giving vasopressin to patients with memory loss resulting from accidental head injuries to aging patients with memory problems. Accident victims suffering amnesia regained their memories and felt more cheerful. Patients with memory problems showed improved attention span, concentration, recall, and ability to learn.

Research on vasopressin provides insight into why people who use recreational drugs often have memory problems. Stimulants like LSD, cocaine, amphetamines, Ritalin, and Cylert cause the pituitary to release vasopressin. Frequent use of these drugs can lead to sluggish mental performance and depression resulting from vasopressin depletion. On the other hand, marijuana and alcohol, which are depressants, inhibit the release of vasopressin. This explains why regular users, especially of marijuana, often complain of memory loss. These problems can be reversed, almost immediately, by inhaling Diapid, because it is absorbed through the mucous membranes in the nose and goes quickly to the brain. Results are often evident in less than a minute. In *High Times* magazine, Dave Brown describes the interaction between vasopressin and marijuana: "A few nasal squirts of this substance can help with the marijuana memory problem, as do other smart drugs, but enough vasopressin will bring one down rather quickly from the high. It is most helpful in relieving some of the herb's sometimes sleepy, cloudy aftereffects."

Additionally, vasopressin can be used to improve memory and recall so that one can learn large amounts of new information. And Pelton reports that it has been remarkably useful in relieving depression.

Diapid, which is a nasal spray manufactured by Sandoz, has been approved by the FDA only to treat the frequent urination associated with diabetes insipidus and bedwetting in children. The FDA has not approved its use in healthy people for memory and learning enhancement. Diapid is considered to be very safe, with no major side effects. However, some people experience mild symptoms such as nose irritation, headaches, abdominal cramps, and an increased desire to move the bowels. Pregnant women should avoid it, since safety during pregnancy has not been established. Soviet studies conducted by Vladimir Frolkis showed that when injected, vasopressin can produce cardiac abnormalities and reduced energy in elderly rats. People with a history of cardiovascular problems should probably not use vasopressin.

Vasopressin can be obtained in the United States by prescription. However, it is poorly reported in the *Physician's Desk Reference* (*PDR*), upon which most physicians rely for prescription information. Few physicians have a working understanding of its uses and effects. It is available over the counter in Mexico. Doses for memory improvement are 12 to 16 USP units a day, or about three to four nasal squirts a day.

Vasopressin is manufactured in three different varieties, each with a slightly different chemical composition. However, the different forms don't appear to have any therapeutic differences. Should you encounter them, the different forms are lysine-vasopressin manufactured by Sandoz in its Diapid Nasal Spray (also known as LVP, Lypressin, Postacton, and Synopressin), arginine-vasopressin (also known as AVP, argipressin, and rinder-vasopressin), and L-desamino-8-D-arginine (also known as DDAVP, Adiuretin SD, DAV Ritter, Desmopressin, Desmospray, and Minirin). They are all nasal sprays.

CENTROPHENOXINE

Commonly known by its trade name, Lucidril, centrophenoxine rejuvenates brain cells and reverses the aging process by getting rid of lipofuscin deposits, which are cellular garbage created by the buildup of toxic waste by-products of cellular metabolism. You might think of centrophenoxine as the "garbage man of the brain." Lipofuscin deposits in the skin are the brown age spots or liver spots commonly seen in older people. Lipofuscin deposits build up in brain cells, causing neurons to die, which results in a decline in mental functioning.

Animal studies indicate an inverse relationship between lipofuscin deposits and learning. That is, the greater the lipofuscin in the brain cells, the less the learning ability; the less lipofuscin, the greater the learning ability. After taking centrophenoxine people report greater alertness and increased feelings of stimulation. Animal studies show improvements in learning.

The rejuvenating effects in humans is believed to be produced by regeneration of parts of the neurons. Centrophenoxine therapy gets rid of the lipofuscin deposits in the brain and skin. Centrophenoxine contributes to intelligence and memory enhancement because it repairs the synapses, where the neurotransmitters are released and pass information.

Centrophenoxine breaks down into dimethylaminoethanol (DMAE) in the blood stream. DMAE is normally found in small quantities in the brain. It is a free-radical scavenger, and has a variety of beneficial brain-boosting effects, including improving mood, intelligence, memory, and learning ability.

Another benefit of centrophenoxine is protection against oxygen starvation or hypoxia. Although the research is scanty, centrophenoxine may benefit conditions where oxygen to brain tissue has been reduced, as in strokes, heart attacks, and drowning. It is known, however, that

---

ALCOHOL IS A MAKE-YOU-STUPID DRUG

Because alcohol is encouraged by our culture, we get the idea that it isn't dangerous. However, alcohol is the most potent and most toxic of the legal psychoactive drugs. It is "harder" than heroin, cocaine, LSD, and many other illegal drugs. Alcohol burns up B vitamins, especially B_1 (thiamine). Andrew Weil recommends that any one who drinks should take 100 mg. on days when drinking to protect the nervous system.

Most people don't know that alcoholic beverages are exempted from labeling requirements. This means they can contain harmful additives that are not listed on the labels. Wines can contain sulfite preservatives and liqueurs may be dyed with artificial colors.

Alcohol poisons the brain and uniformly depresses brain function. The first area to be affected by alcohol is the limbic or emotional area of the brain.

Chronic alcohol abuse can produce memory loss in many ways. For example, focusing of attention becomes more difficult, speed of learning is slowed down, and the rate of forgetting of new memory is increased. The retrieval of memories is also slowed down, and reconstructing memories is more difficult. In fact, all intellectual functions are diminished to some degree. People who drink steadily over a period of hours or days can be left with blank spots in their memories during the the period of their intoxication, which is sometimes called the Lost Weekend.

---

centrophenoxine stimulates energy production. The uptake of glucose or sugar, which is essential for energy production, is increased by centrophenoxine. In the process of producing energy, oxygen is consumed and carbon dioxide created as a by-product. Both oxygen consumption and CO_2 production are increased by centrophenoxine.

Centrophenoxine has some contraindications. In rare cases, people using it experience headaches, muscle stiffness, and excitability. The side effects are similar to those experienced by people taking too much of the nutrient choline. These symptoms are eliminated by reducing the dosage. People on an anti-cholinergic diet should not use centrophenoxine. Centrophenoxine is not currently available in the U.S. It is sold in Europe, however.

FIPEXIDE

So far, little is known about the effects of this cognitive enhancer, which is also known by the names Attentil, BP 662, and Vigilor. In the few tests that have been done with elderly people with cognition disorders, fipexide has been found to improve cognition, short-term memory, and attention. Scientists working with animals have found that those given fipexide before they were exposed to new tasks learned faster. Whereas most nootropics improve both learning and recall, fipexide helps learning but not recall.

Nootropics in the pyrrolidone family work by affecting the parts of the nervous system that use acetylcholine as a neurotransmitter. Fipexide works by slightly increasing the amount of the neurotransmitter dopamine, in the brain. With more dopamine, there is better motor coordination, an improved immune system, more motivation to act, and a better emotional balance, all of which might contribute to the kind of mental fine tuning that promotes learning. The general dose is 200 mg. three times a day.

VINPOCETINE

Sometimes called Cavinton, Vinpocetine is derived from vincamine, which is an extract of the periwinkle plant. It has a very powerful stimulating effect on memory. Vinpocetine ups the metabolism in the brain in four ways. It pumps up the blood flow, increases the rate at which brain cells produce ATP (which is a cell molecule that creates energy), and speeds up the use of glucose and oxygen in the brain. The result is that the cells of the brain can better retain information; so the individual can remember more. Because of its stimulating effect on blood flow, vinpocetine has been used to treat circulatory problems in the brain and memory problems due to low circulation.

Gedeon Richter, a Hungarian company that markets vinpocetine in Europe, has funded more than a hundred studies to show its effectiveness and safety. Many of these studies have shown the drug's powerful effect on memory improvement. In one study, people who had cerebral insufficiency were able to remember more words after being treated. They could recall only six out of ten on a list in the beginning, whereas after using vinpocetine most patients remembered all the words on the list. In another test with normal volunteers, the results showed a dramatic increase in memory on a short-term memory test. Volunteers had to indicate whether three numbers they saw on a computer screen turned up in a long string of numbers they were shown subsequently. Subjects could do this much more quickly after taking a small amount of vinpocetine. The amount of time may not sound like much to a lay person, since the response time was measured in milliseconds—450 milliseconds to 700 milliseconds to respond. But to a scientist, the increase is over 50 percent, contributing to the conclusion that this is a powerful memory improver that is generally very safe. Vinpocetine is not toxic and is considered safe. Typically, people take 5 to 10 mg. a day. It takes about a year of daily use to achieve maximum effect.

• • •

This chapter reviews the most popular nootropics, how they are used as cognitive enhancers, as well as what ailments they can be prescribed to treat. While this book explores what drugs might be used for what purposes, it is not meant to be a guide for obtaining smart drugs. The directory of doctors in Appendix A may help readers find a sympathetic physician. Appendix B lists several suppliers of pharmaceuticals and vitamins that can also serve as a starting point for ordering products by mail. Readers who wish to learn the ins and outs of obtaining smart drugs should also consult *Smart Drugs & Nutrients* by Ward Dean, M.D., and John Morgenthaler, who maintain a list of knowledgeable physicians and keep abreast of the FDA policies. Another helpful source is *Drugs Available Abroad*, an easily accessible guide, with addresses and contact information to a thousand foreign pharmaceuticals, published by Gale Research.

The nootropic smart drugs are gentle, low-key learning and memory enhancers without other effects on the central nervous system. There are, however, more powerful brain boosters that have a more potent impact on the chemistry of the body as a whole, as well as on intelligence, memory, and learning. Again, there is disagreement as to whether a particular substance is to be considered a drug or a nutrient, but we'll use the general consensus in the field and the decisions of the FDA in classifying substances as drugs. According to Michael Hutchinson and John Morgenthaler, writing in *Potential Brain-Food and Mind-Machine Interactions,* more than thirty chemicals have been found to improve either human or animal intelligence or both.

8

OTHER BRAIN-CELL REJUVENATORS

THE MAO INHIBITORS

Monoamine neurotransmitters are chemicals in the synapses that promote feelings of well-being and alertness and increase energy levels. They include dopamine, serotonin, and norepinephrine. With aging, levels of these "feel good" brain chemicals decline, and inadequate amounts can result in depression.

Monoamine oxidase (MAO) is an enzyme that oxidizes monoamine neurotransmitters, including L-dopa and dopamine. With age, MAO levels in the brain increase. MAO inhibitors are drugs that block the action of MAO in the brain and the body. As MAO levels are reduced, feelings of well-being and high energy return.

DEPRENYL

There are two types of MAO. MAO A is found in most body tissues, and MAO B is found primarily in the brain, in the cells around the neurons. Some MAO inhibitors inhibit both types, which can push levels of MAO activity down too far. If MAO activity is decreased too much, the body can end up with too many monoamines, which over-stimulates the neurons and is like being "hyped up" on amphetamines.

L-Deprenyl, sold in the United States as Eldepryl, avoids the danger of hyperstimulation by inhibiting only the type-B MAO in the brain.

According to Steven Fowkes, editor of *Smart Drug News,* published by the Cognitive Enhancement Research Institute, deprenyl is the only MAO B inhibitor in clinical use today.

Deprenyl was discovered in the 1950s and researched extensively by Dr. Joseph Knoll, a Hungarian pharmacologist. Deprenyl is a derivative of phenethylamine (PEA), which is contained in chocolate and might be considered a kind of "love chemical," because people in love have above-average amounts of it in their brains. Deprenyl contributes to both increased sex drive and longevity. It has been shown to quite significantly extend the lives of rats, as well as to increase their sexual activity (measured in "mounting frequency"). It even revitalizes the sex lives of older rats which had ceased to be sexually active. These facts may make deprenyl the first scientifically confirmed aphrodisiac. Fowkes predicts that deprenyl may one day "make sexually active centenarians commonplace."

Deprenyl is also chemically related to amphetamine, which stimulates the brain to release certain neurotransmitters, including dopamine. Deprenyl works by inhibiting the type-B MAO in the brain, and helps increase the neurotransmitter dopamine in the brain. Deprenyl works by increasing the enzymes superoxide dismutase (SOD) and catalase. These enzymes are important because they retard oxidation of neurons and neurotransmitters like dopamine. Oxidation has a damaging impact, because it not only destroys the neurons being oxidized but creates free radicals as a by-product. Free radicals slow down brain functioning and cause symptoms of mental impairment, such as Parkinsonism. The decline is compounded by the fact that dopamine production decreases with age, especially after 45.

Deprenyl's ability to slow the progression of Parkinson's disease and extend the life-span of Parkinson's patients is nearly miraculous. Some scientists believe that regular use of deprenyl prior to the onset of Parkinson's symptoms can prevent the disease entirely.

The same neurons destroyed in Parkinson's disease are destroyed naturally in the course of aging. However, in Parkinson's the rate of destruction is greatly accelerated. Dr. Knoll's research strongly suggests that long-term treatment with Deprenyl can slow the aging process in normal people.

WITH DEPRENYL OLD DOGS *CAN* LEARN NEW TRICKS

Old dogs can suffer from a dementia that is similar to that suffered by humans. They no longer recognize familiar people, wander around aimlessly, and sometimes lose bladder control. Deprenyl Animal Health, Inc., a small company in Overland, Kansas, patented a drug based upon L-Deprenyl as a treatment for senile dogs. David Bruyette, assistant professor at the College of Veterinary Medicine at Kansas State University, studied its effect on three senile dogs. After treatment most of the dogs' symptoms receded, and they returned to normal behavior. Use of deprenyl with dogs is in such an early stage that it is unknown how long the improvements last. Bruyette said that in humans there can be very good results right after treatment, but then the effect eventually disappears. Patent #5,151,449.

People do take deprenyl for life-extension purposes. Dr. Knoll recommends that people forty-five years old take 5 mg. of deprenyl three times a week. The Life Extension Foundation cautions in *The Physician's Guide to Life Extension Drugs* that higher doses are less effective and can have undesirable side effects. They further urge that life-extension therapy with deprenyl should be under the guidance of a qualified physician.

In low doses, people using deprenyl report mild feelings of being generally more alert, with increased energy, a greater sense of well-being, a higher sex drive, and increased assertiveness. However, too much can lead to feeling overstimulated and "speedy." It is important to not take too much, and to increase dosages only gradually to achieve an optimum effect.

Clinical uses of deprenyl are to alleviate depression, increase motor control, reduce muscle ticks, and stimulate sex drive, especially in those over forty-five years of age. Dr. Knoll recommends 5 mg. three times a week for healthy adults. For antidepressant and aphrodisiac use, 1 to 5 mg. are taken daily for thirty days. The antidepressant effects are enhanced by taking 250 mg. of the amino acid L-phenylalanine at the same time.

A growing body of research points to deprenyl as a promising treatment for Alzheimer's disease. With age, there is a progressive increase in MAO B levels in the normal brain. Alzheimer's patients have even higher levels of MAO B than healthy elderly people. Since MAO oxidizes dopamine and other neurotransmitters, there seems to be an acceleration in the degradation of dopamine, norepinephrine, and phenylethlamine, with a resulting dramatic decline in memory, movement, sex drive, and coordination. When Alzheimer's sufferers were given 10 mg. of deprenyl daily, there was a substantial reduction in oxidation of these vital brain chemicals. Alzheimer's sufferers treated with deprenyl demonstrate significant improvements in cognitive behavior and neuroendocrine function with few side effects. Anxiety, depression, and conceptual disorganization decrease, and verbal communication and optimism increase. Alzheimer's patients concentrate, learn, and remember better when taking deprenyl. More is not better, however. Patients receiving 40 mg. per day of deprenyl (which is a very large dose) show less progress and greater side effects.

When the cerebrospinal fluid of Alzheimer's patients using 10 mg. per day of deprenyl was analyzed, there were significant changes in neurotransmitter metabolites in the fluid, which confirmed that MAO B had been inhibited. Further research demonstrated that deprenyl was more effective in treating Alzheimer's than was tranylcypromine, which inhibits both MAO A and MAO B.

Despite these results, the FDA has not approved deprenyl for treating Alzheimer's disease. The only approved use of deprenyl is for treating Parkinson's disease. It is unlikely that deprenyl will be approved for treating Alzheimer's any time soon, because the approval process is so costly. It is estimated to average $231 million to meet the requirements for new drug approval.

Medical doctors can prescribe deprenyl to Alzheimer's patients, but few do so. There are several reasons for this, according to Saul Kent, publisher of the *Life Extension Report*. First, only a minority of doctors know about research on deprenyl as a treatment for Alzheimer's and its encouraging results. Further, pharmaceutical companies are prohibited by the FDA under the labeling regulations from disseminating information about treating Alzheimer's with deprenyl. To do so they must first get the use "approved"—so it is something of a Catch-22. Doctors are further dissuaded from prescribing deprenyl for Alzheimer's by worry about the risk of a malpractice suit for prescribing a drug for an unapproved use. Finally, health-insurance companies won't pay for unapproved treatments.

HYPOTHYROIDISM OR ALZHEIMER'S

Hypothyroidism can be misdiagnosed as Alzheimer's disease. Hypothyroidism is easy to treat and reversible. No one should be diagnosed as having Alzheimer's disease before a complete blood and urine evaluation is made by appropriate laboratory studies. Chemical analysis of the blood should always include a thorough check of thyroid function, as well as measures of the effectiveness of the liver, kidneys, and the other endocrine glands as well. Today dementia and memory loss produced by abnormalities of the thyroid, adrenal cortex, insulin-secreting glands in the pancreas, parathyroid, and pituitary are too easy to diagnose and treat to allow any of them to cause memory loss and mental deterioration.

Vernon Mark and Jeffrey Mark
Reversing Memory Loss

Increasingly, families of Alzheimer's sufferers are educating themselves and joining support organizations. They seek out receptive doctors and educate them. William Summers, a psychiatrist in Arcadia, California, has organized an Alzheimer's Buyer's Club that sells deprenyl by mail order from Costa Rica.

DIMETHYLAMINOETHANOL (DMAE)

Depending on how it is packaged, dimethylaminoethanol (DMAE) can be considered a drug or a nutrient. It is naturally present in small amounts in the human brain, and is found in certain seafoods, including sardines and anchovies, in which it is considered a food or nutrient.

DMAE has much the same effects as centrophenoxine or Lucidril. It increases intelligence, memory, and learning abilities, as well as producing a better mood and more energy. DMAE is a central-nervous-system stimulant and has an uplifting effect similar to that of amphetamines, without the "rush" and subsequent let down or "crash." In small doses it has a milder, continuing effect. During the first two weeks of use, the stimulating effect gradually builds up. People report that mood elevation is continually present. When discontinued, people report no depression or other letdown.

Laboratory studies have shown that older adults suffering from memory loss have decreased levels of acetylcholine. Low levels of acetylcholine have been linked to neurological and learning problems. DMAE stimulates the production of choline, which then helps the brain better produce acetylcholine. Acetylcholine improves ability to think and learn, because it is the main neurotransmitter that promotes memory and learning. The effect that DMAE has on the production of acetylcholine is increased by taking it with vitamin B_5 and calcium panthothenate.

When Riker marketed Deaner, a drug closely related to DMAE, it was described as helping people with learning and memory problems, including a reduced attention span, difficulties with reading and speech, and a lowered achievement level, as well as help with movement and behavior problems. Even though it was considered to be very safe, Deaner was taken off the market in 1983 after the FDA required efficacy studies to prove its effectiveness. Market demands did not justify the cost of the needed clinical trials so Deaner was discontinued.

Deaner is available in Europe under the name Deanol-Riker. The generally recommended dose for cognitive enhancement is 400 mg. per day. However, experimentation under the guidance of a physician may be necessary to establish the optimal dose for any particular individual. Except in very sensitive people, full therapeutic benefits are seen only after several weeks of use. Starting with a small dose is always advisable. Deaner should not be taken by anyone with epilepsy or a history of convulsions. Some people experience mild headaches, weight loss, and insomnia. These symptoms are usually mild and short term. They can be eliminated by reducing the dose.

However, DMAE is still available as a nutritional supplement, which is a milder and safer stimulant. People using it report feeling better, having more energy, and thinking, learning, and remembering more. As a nutrient, it is available in many forms such as bulk powder, capsules, and liquid. Trade names include Acumen, Atrol, Bimanol, Cervoxan, Diforene, Dimethaen, dimethylaminoethanol, Elevan, Pabenol, Paxanol, Risatarun, Tonibral, Varesal, and DMAE-H3.

PHENYTOIN OR DILANTIN

Phenytoin is a remarkable multipurpose drug that has been the subject of more than 8,000 published papers. It is the most common treatment for epilepsy, and is prescribed under the generic name phenytoin and its trade name, Dilantin. It normalizes and improves mental functioning in general and improves concentration, learning, and thinking in particular.

Discovered in 1938, phenytoin was used as an anticonvulsant and is still heralded as the most effective drug for this purpose ever discovered. Although scientists are just beginning to understand the electrical nature of humans and other animals, most people know that our nerves are electrical in nature. Thinking, memory, and pain are all electrically generated. Phenytoin stabilizes the electrical activity in the body at the level of the cell membrane. Dr. Pelton says, "It doesn't matter what area of the body is afflicted, when any area is out of balance electrically, phenytoin can help to normalize the malfunction." Phenytoin stops convulsions, which are electrical in nature. When cells show too much or too little electrical activity, phenytoin brings them back into balance. In addition, when the brain cells are functioning normally, the drug can calm the individual and increase energy levels. So phenytoin acts as a kind of medical equivalent to meditation, promoting calm and harmony.

Because phenytoin influences electric currents, it can affect thinking and recall. Scientists don't really understand how phenytoin works; however, they postulate that it influences electromagnetic fields, which polarize the electrically charged elements in the cells. This results in a more effective organizational structure, so that cell and brain functioning is improved.

One of the major advantages of phenytoin is it stabilizes and normalizes the nervous system without acting as either a stimulant or a depressant. The result is that one can concentrate, learn, and remember better. For example, it is difficult to concentrate while dozens of thoughts are racing through your mind. You are drawn in too many directions. People with such concentration problems report that when taking phenytoin, they can more easily focus their attention. For example, college students with concentration problems reported being less tired and made fewer errors after they used phenytoin. Research on normal healthy adults of various ages has demonstrated that those taking phenytoin have showed improvements in long-term memory, comprehension, learning new material, and intelligence scores.

Prolonged concentration can be exhausting. One effect of phenytoin is that it delays the onset of fatigue and thereby reduces errors that accompany fatigue. In this regard, phenytoin's effect is similar to that of stimulants, but it is not a stimulant and has none of the side effects common to stimulants.

A number of studies using I.Q. tests as a standard have shown significant improvement in scores after using phenytoin. This apparent

NERVE-GROWTH FACTORS

In an important sense, our brains can keep right on growing, and even repairing themselves to some extent when
they get out of kilter. In the 1960s and 1970s, researchers
at Cambridge University in England and the University of
Rochester in the United States found that as they get older
or become damaged, some brain cells actually send out
new "branches"—long, spidery projections called *dendrites*. These dendrites continue to grow longer and sprout
more branches even as we pass our ninetieth birthdays,
leading some experts to speculate that these dendritic
branches are the physical embodiments of what we call the
"wisdom of age."

Recently, scientists have discovered clues that dendritic
branching is stimulated by powerful brain chemicals known
as nerve growth factors (NGF). These chemicals—there
may be dozens or even hundreds of them—are generating
tremendous excitement in laboratories here and abroad.

At the University of Lund in Sweden, Anders Bjorklund
immerses elderly rats in a Morris maze—a tank filled with
murky water that hides a submerged platform. Once the
rat can find the platform and scramble onto it, it's raised
out of the water to safety. As far as the rat is concerned,
the trick is to find the platform during the first immersion,
then remember where it is on subsequent dunkings. The
bottom line on this experiment is that rats who got injections of nerve-growth factor after their first immersion
remembered where the platform was and swam for it, while
rats who got no nerve-growth factor floundered around the
tank until they stumbled on the platform by accident. Obviously, nerve-growth factor has a positive, and possibly life-
saving, impact on the rats' memories.

Kathy Keeton
Longevity: The Science of Staying Young

improved I.Q. is a result of phenytoin's beneficial impact on concentration and general thinking.

Generally phenytoin's effectiveness for a wide variety of disorders is unknown to most doctors. Most doctors think it is useful only in maintaining epilepsy, and are not knowledgeable about its tremendous impact on general cognitive functioning, mood moderation, and concentration.

Phenytoin does have some significant but infrequent side effects when taken in regular dosages. Some people report tremors, insomnia, headaches, dizziness, nausea, and vomiting. Dr. Pelton indicates that phenytoin can occasionally cause liver toxicity during the first few weeks of use. Some people, mostly children with epilepsy, report gum problems.

A major consideration for most people using phenytoin is that it can disturb absorption of vitamin D and folic acid, which are essential for health. Dr. Pelton recommends that people on phenytoin therapy take supplements of vitamin D, calcium, and folic acid. Doses of 25 to 50 mg. per day are generally recommended for cognitive enhancement.

Phenytoin is available, by prescription, in capsule, tablet, and liquid forms. The original patent has expired; so it is available under its generic name, phenytoin, as well as under its trade name Dilantin in the United States, and Epanutin, Epamin, Eplin, Idantoin, and Aleviatan in other countries.

DEHYDROEPIANDROSTERONE (DHEA)

Relatively little is known yet about dehydroepiandrosterone (DHEA), which is a steroid hormone produced by the adrenal glands. It's actually the most common steroid in the blood, and combats aging, obesity, tumors, and cancer. Early research suggests that it protects the brain cells from various conditions associated with aging, such as Alzheimer's disease, mental degeneration, and senility.

Normal brain tissue contains 6.5 times more DHEA than other bodily tissue. As people age, the amount of DHEA in the blood drops, which contributes to loss of mental functioning. According to Dean and

Morgenthaler, research suggests that adding DHEA to nerve cells can halt or reverse age-related decline and even improve functioning. They report a study by Dr. Eugene Roberts, who found that when a small amount of DHEA was added to cultures of nerve cells, there was an increase in the number of neurons and in their connections. Also, DHEA has been found to improve the ability of mice to remember things longer.

Because of the paucity of research, DHEA's use is definitely experimental. It has not been approved by the FDA and is not available by prescription. Researchers are trying to learn how it affects humans, particularly when used on a long-term basis. However, it has recently gained a great deal of attention because it is believed to improve the immune system and protect against viruses. People with AIDS have been using it. There is little in the medical literature about the results of the self-treatment by AIDS sufferers. They have managed to by-pass the medical establishment by going through nonprofit "buyer's clubs" that import DHEA and other drugs into the United States for personal use. The optimal dosage of DHEA in humans is unknown. Dr. Ward Dean recommends in *Smart Drugs & Nutrients*, which he co-authored with John Morgenthaler, that persons using DHEA have their blood levels of DHEA clinically tested every few months. Doses can be increased gradually until blood level tests match that of a twenty year old.

DHEA is available outside the U.S. as Astenile, Deandros, dehydroepiandrosterone, dehyrdoisoandrosterone, Diandron, Prasterone, Psicosterone, and trans-dehydroandrosterone.

TACRINE OR THA

Tacrine or THA (tetrahydroaminoacridine) has been demonstrated in research by Dr. Mohs and by Dr. Summers to consistently improve memory in Alzheimer's patients. It is believed that Alzheimer's is caused, in part, by the body's inability to make enough acetylcholine, which is an important neurotransmitter. After a message is transmitted, another chemical called cholinesterase is used by cells receiving the message to dispose of excess acetylcholine. According to Thomas Donaldson in *Life Extension Report,* THA interferes with this disposal process, which helps people whose memory problems stem from too little acetylcholine.

Dr. Summers has had very hopeful results treating Alzheimer's with a combination of deprenyl and THA plus the nutrient lecithin. Deprenyl increases availability of the neurotransmitters dopamine, norepinephrine, and phenylethylamine, which play a critical role in motor, behavior, and cognitive functions. THA helps to preserve acetylcholine in the brain, and lecithin is a nutrient from which the body manufactures acetylcholine. Although deprenyl and THA plus lecithin work according to different mechanisms, it is believed the combination of the two is more effective in improving memory in Alzheimer's patients.

Summers used THA plus lecithin extensively with patients with good success until July 1990, when the FDA forced him to stop his project. Unfortunately, THA is hard to obtain, and deprenyl has been approved only for treating Parkinson's disease. As a result, research into improving this treatment is slow, and approval doesn't look likely, which has lead to an outcry by Summers and the families of Alzheimer's sufferers. In 1991, they filed a class-action suit against the FDA. Under pressure from the lawsuit, the FDA decided to allow "expanded access" to THA under its "treatment IND program." However, Saul Kent, publisher of *Life Extension Report,* points out that the promised access is, in fact, limited by many restrictions. As an alternative, Summers's group established an Alzheimer's Buyer's Club in Costa Rica.

GEROVITAL OR GH-3

Dr. Ana Aslan, director of the Institute of Geriatrics in Romania, developed Gerovital (GH-3) in the early 1950s. It rapidly became one of the most popular rejuvenation treatments, with movie stars, world leaders, and politicians, including Mao Tse-Tung, Charles de Gaulle, Ho Chi Minh, Winston Churchill, John F. Kennedy, and even, according to news reports, Ronald Reagan, traveling to Dr. Aslan's clinic for treatment. So many Hollywood stars, including Kirk Douglas, Lena Horne, Lillian Gish, Marlene Dietrich, Charles Bronson, Charlie Chaplin, and Greta Garbo, went to Romania for GH-3 treatment that *60 Minutes* did an on-location special. GH-3 has been hailed as a miraculous youth formula that combats the ravages of aging and makes people feel more energetic and youthful. It is claimed to reverse the aging process, and to improve thinking and memory by providing the nutrients needed to repair damaged cells and membranes.

Cell membranes are a thin layer of fats and proteins that bound the cell body. Procaine hydrochloride can pass through the damaged membranes of diseased cells. It increases the cell's consumption of oxygen, and provides nutrients that help the damaged cells repair or renew membranes. This regeneration helps normalize the chemical balance in the cell and speeds up chemical reactions inside the cells. The DNA level in the cells rises, and proteins are made more quickly. As a result, it is believed, cell functions improve, and the symptoms of disease start to alleviate.

Chemically, GH-3, which is an injectable treatment, is made of procaine hydrochloride mixed with potassium metabisulfate, disodium phosphate, and benzoic acid. Procaine breaks down in the body into PABA (paraminobenzoic acid), a B vitamin, and DEAE (diethylamino-ethanol), which is chemically similar to DMAE and is converted in the cells into choline.

PABA aids the body in blood-cell formation, protein metabolism, and skin functions. A deficiency of PABA can cause constipation, depression, digestive disorders, stress, infertility, fatigue, gray hair, headaches, and irritability. PABA stimulates the intestinal bacterial system to produce the B vitamins folic acid, pantothenic, and biotin, and vitamin K. PABA is rapidly disposed of by the liver; so ingesting it alone can get disappointing results. However, when combined with the procaine hydrochloride molecule, PABA is more effective.

DEAE has an antidepressant effect. Studies at Princeton showed DEAE produces mental stimulation and mild euphoria. DEAE comprises choline and acetylcholine, which make up important neurotransmitters that facilitate brain functioning.

Ana Aslan experimented with the rejuvenative effects of procaine through the late 1940s and well into the 1950s. Out of this research she developed an improved formula, in which she buffered and stabilized the basic procaine hydrochloride, which she called Gerovital H-3 or GH-3. Dr. Aslan presented her results from treatment of more than 2,500 people using GH-3 to the Karlsruhe Therapy Congress. She claimed GH-3 relieved depression, arthritis, angina pectoris, and hypertension, produced muscular vigor, and had a rejuvenative effect at the cellular level. Her results were confirmed in the 1970s on 15,000 people aged 40 to 62.

People taking GH-3 claim relief from a host of ailments and pains. They say it is an antidepressant and brain tonic that makes people more alert and cheerful. It is reported to arrest aging symptoms, hair loss, graying, wrinkling, and hardened skin.

Depression in the elderly was researched by an NIMH team, who concluded that it was caused by a buildup of the enzyme monoamine oxidase (MAO) in the brain. Typically this process begins around age 45 and continues with age.

Dr. Alfred Sapse, who had interned under Ana Aslan, showed that GH-3 is an MAO inhibitor that gave rapid improvement in depression and insomnia patients. They also reported a general improved sense of well-being. Patients with high cholesterol showed reduced serum cholesterol after four weeks' treatment. Sapse's results were replicated at UCLA and Duke University.

Even though numerous impressive studies were conducted in the United States, Sapse was frustrated in his many attempts to gain FDA approval to market GH-3 in the United States as a treatment for depression and aging.

The *Physician's Guide to Life Extension Drugs* cautions that GH-3 and similar formulations should not be taken by people using sulphonamide drugs or combinations such as cotrimoxazole. Neither should it be taken by people who are allergic to procaine or are taking sulfa drugs or MAO inhibitors, by pregnant or lactating women, or by children. They state that there have been no clinical reports of serious acute or chronic reactions to Gerovital therapy, because both PABA and DEAE are rapidly excreted from the body.

EXERCISE AS "ANTI-AGING DRUG"

Exercise has been claimed to be the best "anti-aging" pill
there is, due to the health enhancing effects which it exerts
on many physiological and biological parameters. Some
beneficial effects of exercise are: (1) increased maximal
oxygen uptake; (2) improved body mass index; (3) reduced
systolic blood pressure; (4) reduced resting heart rate;
(5) reduced platelet aggregability; (6) improved glucose
tolerance; (7) reduced insulin resistance; (8) reduced total
cholesterol and triglycerides, and raised HDL cholesterol;
(9) reduced incidence of coronary heart disease; and
(10) reduced incidence of mortality due to all causes. With
such a wide range of positive effects, it is little wonder that
several investigators have also confirmed that exercise also
dramatically reduces biological age.

Vladimir Dilman and Ward Dean
The Neuroendocrine Theory of Aging and
Degenerative Disease

Kathy Keeton, author of *Longevity: The Science of Staying Young*,
discusses Gerovital briefly, stating that her father took it with good
results. But a study conducted at the Los Angeles VA Hospital in the
mid-1970s concluded that there was little scientific basis for Ana
Aslan's claims. Consequently, GH-3 has not been approved for use by
the FDA. Keeton laments, "Sadly, we will probably never know how
effective Dr. Aslan's Gerovital really is, because no drug company will
undertake the enormous expense necessary to prove the worth of the
drug."

The Dr. Ana Aslan Institute in Miami, Florida, provides treatment
using Aslan's original formula. The treatment consists of Gerovital
administered by injection three times a week for four weeks, followed
by a ten-day rest period and another four-week treatment period. GH-

3 also comes in tablet form. The dose is one tablet a day for twenty-five days, then no GH-3 for a five-day "rest" period.

VITACEL

More recently, Dr. Robert Koch, a Salt Lake City biochemist, developed Vitacel 3, which is GH-3 in tableted form and contains the same PBN factor that is the active component of Aslan's injectable GH-3. His formula, Vitacel 4, expands the nutritional benefits of Vitacel 3 by adding bee propolis, which has antibacterial and antiviral activity, and royal jelly, which contains high concentrations of natural pantothenic acid (B_5), vitamin B_6, and vitamin C.

Vitacel 7 is Koch's latest development. It has vitamin-complexing agents that replace the bisulfite and benzoic acid that Dr. Aslan used in GH-3 because they may be possible allergens for some people. Koch claims that this new formulation keeps the procaine hydrochloride working for many hours in the body.

Like GH-3, Vitacel has not been approved by the FDA, and is not available in the United States. However, people are allowed to purchase it offshore, such as in the Cayman Islands, in small quantities for personal use. In this day and age of faxes, people can fax orders or call an 800 toll-free phone number, use a Mastercard or Visa number, and receive Vitacel in the mail in about ten days. One such company is Nutritional Engineering in Grand Cayman in the British West Indies.

K.H.3

Another procaine formulation is K.H.3, which is a gelatine capsule containing procaine and hematoporphyrin. Hematoporphyrin boosts the procaine action. It is claimed to help alertness, concentration, and recall as well as improve a number of health problems. The *Physician's Guide to Life Extension Drugs* reviews many impressive studies showing the effectiveness of K.H.3. The benefits are attributed to improved circulation to the brain. The only state where K.H.3 is sold legally is Nevada. It is also available over the counter in Europe. The dose is one or two capsules a day with food for five months, followed by a two- to

HOW TO ASK YOUR DOCTOR FOR A PRESCRIPTION

Arm yourself with knowledge about the drugs you want that may be beneficial. Buy yourself a copy of the *Physician's Desk Reference*. Your doctor already has a copy of this book, and trusts it. However, the *PDR* does not contain information about non-FDA-approved uses of these drugs. If you want to obtain such information to convince your doctor to prescribe it for you, you'll need to look up some of the literature references given in the bibliography of *Smart Drugs & Nutrients*, *Life Extension* or in this book. You can get copies of these papers in any large medical or life-sciences library.

Don't expect your doctor to know about life-extension uses of prescribed drugs approved for other uses or to be familiar with the research papers you may show him. The pharmaceutical companies are legally prohibited from informing physicians of such non-FDA-approved uses. With the literature you have collected, however, you can demonstrate that (1) the drug you want is low in toxicity and you know how to use it, and (2) you intend to use the drugs in a responsible manner.

If your physician says no to one of your prescription requests, you should be neither angry nor cowed. Ask for an explanation of the objections. In some cases, you will find that the objections are valid. In other cases, the objections will be based on lack of knowledge of the new non-FDA-approved uses for old drugs. Then you should give your doctor copies of the relevant papers. Your doctor is apt to be extremely busy, so don't just give him the literature citation; it is your responsibility to provide full copies of these scientific papers.

Keep the magnitude of your request within reason. You should make it clear that you recognize that your physician's time is valuable and that you are prepared to pay for it, even if it merely involves his or her reading a research paper. There is no such thing as a free lunch.

> Durk Pearson and Sandy Shaw
> *Life Extension*

four-week rest period of no K.H.3. It should not be taken with sulfa drugs or MAO inhibitors, by pregnant or nursing women, or by people allergic to procaine.

OBTAINING THE SMART PHARMACEUTICALS

Although there are a vast and growing number of smart drugs, they are not readily available in the United States, because they have not been approved by the FDA for improving cognition. Some are, however, available by prescription for other uses. The dilemma stems from the fact that the FDA has no category for drugs that are designed strictly to improve cognition in normal, healthy people. The FDA policy is to approve only those drugs known to treat specific diseases such as Alzheimer's disease or senility. To the FDA, the idea of normal, healthy people using drugs to enhance cognition or expand perception is akin to quackery. Consequently, most nootropics designed specifically for cognitive enhancement are not currently approved for use in the U.S. at all.

Many people have been able to get prescriptions easily for nootropics and other smart drugs from doctors in Europe. In the United States, however, it is not so easy. Prescriptions for smart drugs are hard to get, because nootropics are not designed to cure an ailment, but to help people think better instead. According to Dean and Morgenthaler, several pharmaceutical companies have attempted, without success, to get FDA approval to sell nootropics and other smart drugs in the U.S.

9

VITAMINS TO BOOST YOUR BRAIN POWER

Old wives' tales about the miracle powers of vitamins abound. Well, it's turning out that a lot of the old wives' tales are true. Although people didn't understand how or why certain foods, such as fish, are good for the brain, they became part of our common wisdom. But the latest research has demonstrated that vitamins can, in fact, increase brain power. This chapter highlights the vitamins that improve thinking, learning, memory, and other cognitive functions of the brain.

THE BRAIN-BOOSTING VITAMINS

Brain-boosting vitamins are the elite among the vitamins we get from foods, supplements, and sources within our own body. Scientists have identified thirteen brain-boosting vitamins. Vitamins are organic substances that help regulate the chemical reactions in the body to protect cells and change food into energy and living tissues. Some vitamins are produced within our own body. Vitamin D, for example, is manufactured by the skin after exposure to sunlight. Vitamin K, biotin, and pantothenic acid are produced in the body by the bacteria in the stomach. Most vitamins, however, are obtained from foods and drinks.

Vitamins are usually divided into two groups: water-soluble vitamins and fat-soluble vitamins. Water-soluble vitamins include B-complex vitamins and vitamin C. Vitamins A, D, and E are fat-soluble.

The body can store fat-soluble vitamins, but water-soluble vitamins must be constantly replenished.

Early nutritionists promoted vitamins to correct deficiency diseases such as scurvy, anemia, and rickets. By the 1970s, researchers had noticed an apparent link between diet and health. People who ate better diets tended to be less likely to get heart disease, cancer, and other diseases. In the 1980s, researchers became aware of the connection between vitamin deficiency and common neurological defects in newborns, such as spina bifida, in which the spinal cord is not properly closed, and anencephaly, where the brain doesn't fully develop.

And now, in the 1990s, researchers are substantiating what "health nuts" have been saying. Optimum quantities of certain vitamins improve brain functioning. The greatest interest surrounds the vitamins that function as antioxidants, which include vitamins C, E, and beta-carotene, the chemical substance that produces vitamin A. What is exciting is that these vitamins can get rid of free radicals, the unstable toxic molecules produced during normal cell metabolism, or when the body is deprived of sufficient oxygen, or when it is exposed to sunlight, x-rays, ozone, tobacco smoke, the fumes from a car, and various environmental pollutants. Free radicals damage DNA, change the biochemical mix in the body, wear down cell membranes, and sometimes actually kill cells. As these damages build up, diseases, such as cancer and heart disease, deterioration from aging, and neurological damage can result. The latest research indicates that vitamins, like knights to the rescue, can help stave off these damages. Antioxidizing vitamins fend off and destroy the rampaging free radicals, thereby enabling people to avoid certain types of cell damage and to experience higher levels of wellness.

Initially, the study of vitamins focused on how they protect against physical damages to the body, such as the possibility that vitamin C prevents cataracts, and that vitamin E prevents heart disease and improves the immune system. More recently, there has been a growing interest in how antioxidant vitamins protect against mental decline and act as brain boosters. The thrust in the '90s is a shift from interest in how to prevent disease and decline of health to developing consumption guidelines for functioning mentally and physically at optimal levels.

BETA-CAROTENE

Beta-carotene has attracted growing attention in brain-boosting research circles. It is found in some fruits and dark-green and orange vegetables, such as spinach, carrots, and sweet potatoes. Beta-carotene is not itself a vitamin. It is a precursor that is converted into vitamin A in the body. After its transformation, it functions as an antioxidant, neutralizing free radicals, which cause damage and contribute to cancer and other serious health problems.

The research on the power of beta-carotene and its alter ego, vitamin A, is impressive. For example, a Boston team of researchers led by Charles Hennekens studied several hundred doctors taking 50 mg. of beta-carotene every other day. They found that the frequency of heart attack, stroke, and death were about half the rate as those who didn't take beta-carotene. Beta-carotene and vitamin A are associated with lower rates of lung cancer and tumors of the mouth and throat. Vitamin A promotes healthy skin, hair, nails, and good vision; improves the functioning of the immune system; and reduces incidences of infections and promotes rapid healing.

Beta-carotene and the vitamin A it produces have been found to have powerful effects on the mind as well. Vitamin A protects brain-cell membranes, which have high concentrations of fat and are easily damaged by the actions of the free radicals. Beta-carotene itself acts as an antioxidant and attacks two of the most damaging free radicals, polyunsaturated fatty-acid radicals and oxygen radicals. Because vitamin A and beta-carotene are fat-soluble antioxidants, they prevent the free radicals from damaging the fatty-cell membranes.

Vitamin A is found in two forms. One is beta-carotene, also called pro-vitamin A, which comes primarily from plant food sources. The other is vitamin A, also called retinol, and comes only from animal food sources, where it exists initially in a preformed state.

A good source of vitamin A is fish liver and fish-liver oils; so the old wives' tale about fish being a brain food is correct. Beef and chicken liver also have high levels of vitamin A. Beta-carotene is found in dark green plants like spinach, broccoli, Swiss chard, kale, and collard greens. Orange plants, such as carrots, sweet potatoes, winter squash, pumpkins, apricots, cantaloupes, mangoes, and papaya, are also high in beta-carotene.

A variety of food supplements provide either vitamin A or beta-carotene in higher concentrations. Vitamin A from fish-liver oil is available in gelatine capsules. Vitamin A can be purchased in health-food stores in a mycelized liquid form, which has been processed to increase the rate of absorption into the body and is over five times as effective as the vitamin A in the oil-based gelatine capsule. Beta-carotene usually comes in a capsule or orange-powder form. Vitamin A and beta-carotene are absorbed more completely if taken with a meal containing fat.

Vitamin A and beta-carotene are often taken together because they each have unique antioxidant properties. The RDA for vitamin A is 5,000 international units. Nutritionists recommend, however, taking more beta-carotene than vitamin A. Beta-carotene is nontoxic. Large amounts may cause a yellowing of the skin, which subsides when intake is reduced. This condition is not harmful; however, taking vitamin A in doses of more than 25,000 international units for prolonged periods can cause headaches, vomiting, and damage to the eyes and liver, which is the primary storage site in the body for vitamin A. During pregnancy, women should take vitamin A only as prescribed by a doctor.

VITAMIN B

Six B vitamins all contribute to good mental functioning. Though different B vitamins may play slightly different roles, they're all part of a complex. According to Dr. Ward Dean and John Morgenthaler, the authors of *Smart Drugs & Nutrients,* if you take one for a specific purpose, it's still a good idea to take the others as well. This is done by taking a B-complex pill or a multiple vitamin with a full B-complex complement. Because the B vitamins are soluble in water and aren't stored in the fat cells, their effect is gone in a few hours; so nutritionists recommend taking a series of doses throughout the day.

VITAMIN B$_1$

Like many of the other brain boosters, vitamin B$_1$, or thiamine, is a strong antioxidant that fights free radicals. Thiamine aids in energy metabolism, appetite maintenance, nervous-system function, and cell repair. John Mann in *Secrets of Life Extension* notes that B$_1$'s main antioxidant protection occurs when it regulates and normalizes oxidative metabolism in the course of transforming glucose to energy. Vitamin B$_1$ can be taken to counteract the negative effects of alcohol oxidation on nerve cells after drinking too much. B$_1$ has been used to treat organic brain dysfunctions, such as "organic brain syndrome," and research suggests that it contributes to better brain functioning in the normal brain as well.

Thiamine is found in pork, bran, whole-grain cereals, soybeans, split peas, lima beans, and sunflower seeds. The RDA for thiamine is 1.5 mg. Mann suggests that most people need between 25 to 100 mg. daily. People do sometimes take higher doses, up to 1,000 mg., to give an energy lift. However, Mann cautions that prolonged use of high doses of thiamine can disrupt the normal B balance and cause deficiencies in other B vitamins. This problem can be avoided if other B vitamins are well-provided by a B-complex supplement.

VITAMIN B$_3$

Vitamin B$_3$, or niacin, helps improve the memory and protect against stress. Niacin reduces blood clotting, which can cause strokes and heart attacks and interfere with brain functioning. Additionally, it improves the oxygen-carrying ability of red blood cells. The more oxygen and blood in the brain, the better the mind works.

Niacin can cause flushing, itching, and skin tingling when taken in doses larger than 50 mg. Mann says that this is harmless but can be annoying and that the effect resolves spontaneously with continued use. Alternatively, the effect can be reduced by taking an aspirin an hour before ingesting the niacin. The RDA for niacin is 18 mg. for men and 13 mg. for women. Because niacin is acidic, people with ulcers should take it with an antacid, such as bicarbonate of soda, to avoid aggravating their condition. People with diabetes and high blood pressure should consult a doctor before using niacin in large doses. It is possible to get enough niacin from your diet, especially from high-protein foods like meat, eggs, and enriched cereals.

XANTHINOL NICOTINATE

Xanthinol nicotinate passes through cell membranes more easily than does niacin. When it enters a cell, metabolism of glucose is speeded up, and ATP (adenosine triphosphate) increases. According to Dean and Morgenthaler, ATP is the basic fuel of life. It is a key molecule in the cellular metabolic reaction. Increasing ATP means more energy for everything, including brain work.

Xanthinol nicotinate is a vasodilator that dilates or expands blood vessels, allowing more blood to flow through them. Although it expands blood vessels all over the body, the increased blood flow in the brain is what plays a key role in increasing brain power. More blood flow to the brain means more oxygen is carried to the brain.

Research confirms xanthinol nicotinate's brain-boosting abilities. For example, in a study by S. Loriaux on normal, healthy elderly adults, comparing the effects of xanthinol nicotinate and niacin, xanthinol nicotinate was far and away much better. Both groups showed short-term memory gains, but those taking xanthinol nicotinate showed improvement in both short-term and long-term memory.

There are some precautions in taking this form of niacin. It can cause some minor reactions, including flushing, headaches, heartburn, muscle cramps, blurred vision, vomiting, diarrhea, itchy skin, rash, or skin-color changes. Normally these symptoms go away as you continue to take it. Pregnant women and nursing mothers should consult a physician before taking xanthinol nicotinate. Its use should be avoided by people with ulcers, cardiovascular conditions, or liver problems.

FOR STRESS RELIEF, AVOID DRUGS: DRINK TEAS
Medical doctors hand out millions of prescriptions for tranquilizing drugs. Like alcohol, most of them are depressants that interfere with mental function and carry strong risks of addiction. The most common are the benzodiazepines, a family that includes such well-known members as diazepam (Valium), chlordiazepoxide (Librium), alprazolam (Xanax), and lorazapam (Ativan). In my opinion, these are all dangerous drugs. Most doctors who prescribe them and most patients who take them do not understand their effects or appreciate their dangers. Benzodiazepine addiction is one of the most difficult forms of drug dependence to treat.

I never prescribe these tranquilizers, but I do recommend a few natural substances. Spearmint and chamomile teas are both mildly relaxing. You can drink as much of them as you want. A stronger remedy is passionflower, made from a plant (*Passiflora incarnata*) native to southeastern United States. Tincture of passionflower is available at herb and health-food stores. The dose is one dropperful in a little water up to four times a day as needed. You may be able to find capsules of the freeze-dried plant as well; take one or two of them one to four times a day as needed. Passionflower is not sedating.

Andrew Weil, M.D,
Natural Health, Natural Medicine

Xanthinol nicotinate goes by numerous names, including Androgeron, Angiomanin, Angiomin, Cafardil, Circulan, Clofamin, Complamex, Complamin, Dacilin, Emodinamin, Jupal, Landrina, Niconicol, Sadamin, SK 331 A, Vasoprin, Vedrin, Xanidil, and Xavin. Such names make it sound more like a drug than a nutrient.

Xanthinol nicotinate cannot be purchased in the United States. It is available, however, in Europe and Canada, and can be purchased by mail order from Switzerland and England. A typical dose is 300 to 600 mg. taken three times a day with meals.

VITAMIN B$_5$

Vitamin B$_5$, also called pantothenic acid, is a powerful antioxidant known for increasing stamina and buffering against stress. It is the substance in royal jelly that extends the life of the queen bee beyond that of the workers. And researchers have found that royal jelly in the diet significantly extends the life of certain lab animals.

Pantothenic acid is essential for converting choline to acetylcholine, a neurotransmitter involved in speeding messages from one nerve cell to another. It is necessary for the body to produce steroid hormones, which are particularly important during times of stress.

Dean and Morgenthaler suggest starting with small doses and working slowly up to larger ones taken three or four times a day. They caution that starting with large doses can cause short-term diarrhea.

VITAMIN B$_6$

Vitamin B$_6$, or pyridoxine, is another antistress agent. It is essential for production of norepinephrine, serotonin, and dopamine, which are neurotransmitters needed for optimal mental functioning. Without B$_6$ your body may not be able to manufacture enough of these neurotransmitters, and mental decline may result. B$_6$ is a key agent in protein metabolism, and has been shown to increase the life spans of mice and fruit flies. Deficiencies can lead to depression and increased risk of cardiovascular disease. The RDA is 2 mg. for men and 1 to 6 mg. for women. It is found in meat, fish, nuts, bananas, potatoes, bran, and dairy products.

Dean and Morgenthaler caution that doses higher than 200 mg. per day should never be taken without a doctor's supervision. More than 500 mg. a day can be toxic, producing difficulty in walking and other central-nervous-system symptoms. People with Parkinson's disease taking L-Dopa should always consult a doctor before using B$_6$.

VITAMIN B$_{12}$

Vitamin B$_{12}$, or cyanocobalamin, is also an antistress agent and is effective in combating fatigue. It helps release energy in foods. Some people claim it is an energy and performance booster for athletes. B$_{12}$ is an essential growth factor necessary for proper maintenance of the brain and nerves. Rats given B$_{12}$ learn faster. Deficiencies of B$_{12}$ are associated with some forms of senile dementia and schizophrenia.

LINK BETWEEN VITAMINS AND MENTAL STATES

The right balance between vitamin B$_{12}$ and folic acid (folate) may be vital as we age. Massachusetts researchers say that finding this balance may provide relief for both depression and dementia.

Over the past two decades, several studies have established a firm link between the vitamins and mental states. Among healthy older people, those with the poorest cognitive functioning were lowest on folic acid and B$_{12}$. Alzheimer's patients with higher folate levels were less affected by the disorder. Folic acid also has been shown to enhance cognitive functioning and even prolong life in the elderly and depressed.

Brain/Mind Bulletin
September 1990

People on vegetarian diets may fail to get enough B$_{12}$, because it is not found in plants. It is found in beef, fish, chicken, and dairy products. One amusing anecdote illustrates the connection between meat, vegetarianism, and the need for B$_{12}$. After ordering fast-food hamburgers, three young men experimented with taking their first intramuscular injections of B$_{12}$. When their hamburgers arrived, they all found that they had completely lost their appetite for them. Because Dilantin depletes B$_{12}$, people using it should consult a physician about taking B$_{12}$ supplements. B$_{12}$ is available in sublingual form, as a nasal applicator, and by injection from a physician. The typical dose is 1 mg. a day. Dean and Morgenthaler caution people with gout to generally avoid B$_{12}$ supplements.

VITAMIN C

Vitamin C, or ascorbic acid, is an antioxidant and a substance used in manufacturing neurotransmitters and nerve cells. Vitamin C has probably gotten its greatest boost to fame from Dr. Linus Pauling, who claims it can prevent the common cold. However, it does much more—so much, in fact, that Durk Pearson and Sandy Shaw regard vitamin C as a kind of miracle drug. Dr. Ross Pelton, author of *Mind Foods and Smart Pills*, supports this opinion.

Vitamin C stimulates the immune system, enabling one to better resist diseases. Terminal cancer patients taking megadoses of vitamin C live longer. It promotes faster wound healing and reduces the amount of cholesterol in the blood. It is a powerful detoxifier and protects against the destructive power of many pollutants. In addition, it protects against heart and blood diseases, reduces anxiety, promotes sleep, and is a natural antihistamine.

We are dependent on vitamin C from outside sources, because the body can't manufacture it. A severe deficiency causes scurvy, and eventually death. Mann points out in *Secrets of Life Extension* that although only a little vitamin C is needed to prevent scurvy, much more is needed for optimal health. The RDA of vitamin C is 45 mg. each day, which is just enough to prevent scurvy. Mann points out that research by the Committee on Animal Nutrition shows that a monkey needs 55 mg. of vitamin C per kilogram of body weight. When this measure is extrapolated to humans, a 150-pound person would need 3,850 mg. of vitamin C each day. Mann blasts the attitude of the medical establishment that sets its standards at the minimum level needed to prevent deficiency.

Most importantly for the subject of this book, vitamin C is a key player in the better-brain sweepstakes. It increases mental alertness and functioning in a variety of ways.

HEALTH IS NOT THE ABSENCE OF SYMPTOMS
Until recently, the attitude of most scientists and nutritionists has been that if there was no scurvy, we were getting
enough vitamin C. The absurdity in this reasoning is that
scurvy is not the initial symptom of ascorbic-acid deficiency. It is the final stage preceding death. Enlightened
physicians and nutritionists now use the term *subclinical
scurvy* to indicate states in which we are getting enough of
the vitamin to avoid symptoms of acute and chronic
scurvy, but not enough to prevent less dramatic disorders.

John Mann
Secrets of Life Extension

Vitamin C is the main antioxidant that circulates in the blood. When
available in sufficient quantity, blood carries it around the body,
washing over the cells to create a bath of protection. Like a martyr for
a good cause, whenever a free radical turns up, a molecule of vitamin
C gives up one of its own electrons to render the free radical ineffective,
like a soldier neutralizing an enemy. According to Pelton, the battle
between vitamin C and free radicals goes on repeatedly, maybe more
than 100,000 or a million times a second, depending on the body's level
of metabolism and the amount of vitamin C. The higher the metabolism
rate and the more vitamin C, the more pitched the battle and the more
radicals destroyed. Unfortunately, with each radical decimated, a
molecule of vitamin C is lost, so the body rapidly loses its supply of
vitamin C. But it's for a good cause, for with each C molecule lost, a cell
is saved.

This process works, because the vitamin C operates like a kind of
pump that Dr. Pelton calls the "vitamin-C pump" to clean up the
cerebrospinal fluids surrounding the brain and spinal cord. The central
nervous system has more unsaturated fats than any other organ in the
body, making it more vulnerable to attack by free radicals and oxidation.
The vitamin-C pump removes vitamin C from the blood as it circulates

to increase the amount of vitamin C in the cerebrospinal fluid ten times. The pump then takes the concentrated vitamin C from the cerebrospinal fluid, and concentrates it tenfold again in the nerve cells around the brain and spinal cord. Pelton says that the vitamin-C bath that protects the brain and spinal cord cells has more than a hundred times as much vitamin C as the other normal body fluids. Like an attacking army, the concentrated vitamin C goes after the free radicals threatening to damage nerve cells. The result is akin to a blood bath—though perhaps it's more appropriate to describe this as a "vitamin-C bath"—in which the vitamin-C soldiers lay down their lives for each free radical destroyed in their attack.

Vitamin C protects against the damaging effects of toxins consumed during smoking and drinking, including nicotine, carbon monoxide, nitrogen oxides and nitric acid gas, cadmium, acetaldehaye, poly-nuclear aromatic hydrocarbons, and N-nitroso compounds. Research has demonstrated that vitamin C destroys toxic substances, much in the same way that it combats the free radicals. A molecule of vitamin C gives up the ghost each time a toxic molecule bites the dust. Because this battle against toxins reduces the level of vitamin C, smokers and alcohol drinkers normally have much lower amounts of vitamin C in their blood serum than do those who don't smoke or drink. If you drink or smoke too much, taking extra vitamin C will help protect you from the damaging effects of the toxins associated with your indulgences, including the kind of muddied and confused thinking that can come from drinking too much.

Another important benefit of vitamin C is its contribution to the proper production and release of several important neurotransmitters in the brain, including dopamine and norepinephrine (also referred to collectively as catecholamine production and release).

Research has shown that vitamin C increases mental thinking ability and intelligence. For example, it was learned that geriatric patients in a British hospital who were experiencing mental confusion didn't have enough vitamin C. When given vitamin-C supplements, they improved dramatically. In another study, students with higher vitamin-C levels scored, on the average, five points higher on I.Q. tests than did students with lower levels of vitamin C. When the students with the low vitamin-C levels were given vitamin-C supplements, their average I.Q. scores went up almost four points, showing the power of vitamin C to improve intelligence.

Green vegetables such as broccoli, spinach, kale, brussel sprouts, cabbage, collards, and mustard greens have high vitamin-C content. Other sources of vitamin C include citrus fruits, pineapples, mangoes, and papaya. Nonetheless, research indicates that most people don't get enough vitamin C from diet alone. Generally, health practitioners concerned about nutrition recommend about 1,000 to 3,000 mg. per day of vitamin C, but most Americans get only about 50 mg. a day. Thus, supplements are usually recommended for the best health and protection from the potential damages to neurotransmitters by free radicals. Mann claims that very high doses of vitamin C can prolong life, delay wrinkling, ward off senility, and prolong youthful vigor.

Supplements are available in a variety of forms. Most common are regular and timed-release tablets. Vitamin C is also available in chewable tablets and powder form. The advantage of using the bulk powder is the inexpensive price. However, the powder is difficult to store, because when exposed to air, the ascorbic acid oxidizes to form a toxic substance called dehydroascorbate. Thus, it's important to mix powdered vitamin C fresh each time.

People with sensitive stomachs can have problems taking vitamin C in pills, which dissolve slowly while concentrating acid in the stomach. Powdered vitamin C can be a good alternative. It can be used as a lemon or vinegar substitute, and sprinkled on fish, vegetables, and salads. Or it can be dissolved in a glass of water to make a thirst-quenching drink.

Vitamin C is available in a variety of preparations. Ascorbic acid, the acidic form, is the most common. Less acidic preparations, calcium ascorbate and sodium ascorbate, are also available. The fat-soluble form of vitamin C, ascorbyl palmitate, is more effective than water-soluble forms as an antioxidant in preventing the peroxidation of lipids and in protecting the heart, brain, and central nervous system from free radicals. Like many other vitamins, vitamin C is available in both natural and synthetic forms. According to Pelton, with the exception of vitamin E, most synthetic vitamins are as effective as the natural ones, and they are cheaper.

Researchers have found that a group of compounds called rutins and bioflavonoids or vitamin P are produced along with vitamin C in nature and increase the effectiveness of vitamin C. Taking the two substances together is generally recommended.

Vitamin C is considered to be very safe, even when taken in high doses of 1,000 to 3,000 mg. daily, which is well above the government RDA of 45 to 60 mg. daily. Vitamin C is safe even in very high doses of 10,000 mg. In fact, vitamin C encourages the production of other enzymes that use vitamin C; so the body can use the extra vitamin C that becomes available. Beyond a certain point, taking extra vitamin C probably won't make much difference in body or mental functioning.

Signs of vitamin C deficiency are bleeding gums and easy bruising. Fatigue, mental sluggishness, depression, low resistance to flus and colds, and slow healing may also signal a deficiency.

Signs of vitamin C saturation include gastritis, gas, and diarrhea, and are relatively minor. These are temporary and can be controlled by reducing the dosage. People taking vitamin C in large doses regularly and who wish to stop should do so gradually over a week or two. Stopping abruptly can lead to lowered resistance until the body adjusts to the lower amounts of vitamin C available.

VITAMIN E

Vitamin E, another powerful antioxidant, is a member of a group of compounds called the tocopherols that come in a variety of forms, identified by eight Greek letters—alpha, beta, gamma, delta, epsilon, zeta, eta, and theta—making vitamin E sound like a kind of fraternity or sorority of vitamins.

According to Pelton, vitamin E is nature's "most potent fat-soluble antioxidant" and plays an important role in protecting the membranes of the brain cells and the structures inside the cell from damage by that biggest killer of cells, free radicals. Since the cells in the brain and skin have a greater percentage of fat than other cells in the body, they need the help of the fat-soluble vitamin E to protect them.

Vitamin E takes up residence in the cell membrane to keep the cell wall from being damaged, a little like a guard in the old castles with moats who stands on the castle wall, keeping the enemy from getting in. In the membrane, vitamin E operates to keep the free radicals from getting through to destroy the neurons it protects. As Pelton puts it, vitamin E serves as a "multipurpose defense mechanism against free-radical damage."

Vitamin E is a good team player in working with other vitamins and substances to increase protection and mental power. Vitamin E works in concert with vitamin A to protect against the damage wreaked by air pollutants, especially from nitrogen oxide and ozone. Experts report that vitamin E is more effective when taken with the mineral selenium. It's kind of the vitamin equivalent of Butch Cassidy and the Sundance Kid.

The oils of nuts, seeds, and soybeans are especially rich in vitamin E, as long as they are unrefined and cold-pressed. Soybeans, fresh wheat germ, wheat germ oil, whole grains, nuts, and seeds found in health-food stores are high in vitamin E. Eggs are a good source, although with eggs there is unwarranted concern about getting too much cholesterol. Vitamin E is concentrated in dark leafy vegetables, like broccoli, brussel sprouts, asparagus, and cabbage.

Vitamin E supplements come in both natural and synthetic forms, with varying combinations of tocopherols. The most commonly available supplements are natural mixed tocopherols, natural vitamin E, synthetic vitamin E, and mycelized vitamin E. The latter is a fat-soluble vitamin broken up into small particles to make it soluble in water. Mycelization helps the body to be better able to absorb vitamin E into the membranes of the cell.

As with other vitamins, there has been controversy over the superiority of the natural versus synthetic forms. Some researchers have found that natural vitamin E seems to be more active, perhaps because the vitamin exists in two mirror-image chemical forms: a right-handed chemical arrangement referred to as *D-tocopherol* and a left-handed arrangement called *L-tocopherol*. For whatever it's worth, the right-handed D version is the only one that occurs in nature (so natural vitamin E is sometimes referred to as D-alpha-tocopherol), whereas both forms can be produced synthetically (so synthetic vitamin E is sometimes called DL-alpha-tocopherol).

Another controversy surrounding vitamin E is its safety in large dosages. Because vitamin E is fat-soluble, it is stored in the body tissues, and there is concern that it can build up to a toxic level. Some evidence suggests that too much can cause stomach upset, including nausea, gas, and diarrhea. Extremely high doses given to laboratory animals produces toxic effects on the adrenal, thyroid, and sex glands. Mann recommends daily doses of 800 to 1,220 IU (International Units are 1 mg. each) taken with meals, and not over 1,600 IU daily. He cautions that people with high blood pressure, overactive thyroid, or heart damage from rheumatic fever should seek supervision of a doctor before taking high doses of vitamin E.

As the years go by, the list of scientifically confirmed health benefits from vitamins continues to grow. In recent years, improved brain functioning has been added to this list. This latest addition only serves to confirm the idea that what is good for our bodies and our overall health is good for our minds as well.

10

NUTRIENTS FOR BETTER BRAIN POWER

Certain nutrients in foods are another source of brain power. The distinction between nutrients, drugs, and vitamins gets especially fuzzy, because nutrients are a kind of catch-all category for those combinations of vitamins, minerals, substances not yet classified as drugs, and food extracts that have been combined to form various products. Brain-nourishing nutrients are available in powders, as "smart drink" mixtures to be added to juice, and nutritional supplements in capsules and tablets. The FDA classifications create a lot of confusion by defining certain nutrient products as drugs or controlled substances.

Taking these difficulties into consideration, nutrients are viewed here as products, not currently classified as drugs, which consist of combinations of vitamins, minerals, herbs, or food substances. Some nutrient formulations are mixed on the spot in the form of the smart drinks served at "smart bars" and "smart cafés" at rave parties. These drinks contain a variety of powdered nutrients mixed with juices in secret recipes. Some smart drinks have been commercially packaged, like those formulated by Durk Pearson and Sandy Shaw, and sold at health fairs and by mail order through multilevel companies specializing in life-extension and brain-boosting products.

SMART BABIES

The research of Columbia University psychologist Warren Meck, Ph.D. and his colleagues on rats suggests that it may be possible to permanently enhance memory by increasing the intake of choline during a baby's development in the womb and in the first few months of life. Their results, which were summarized in *Psychology Today*, show that choline produces long-lasting biochemical changes in developing nerve cells, boosts memory function and precision above normal levels, and stalls age-related decline in memory. The results have been so dramatic that Meck believes that choline supplementation may also have a robust effect on human babies.

Where and how supplemental choline acts on the brain is not known. Meck thinks it may trigger increases in nerve growth factor, which helps neurons generate and regenerate and delays the brain cell damage associated with aging. Another theory is that choline restructures the neurons, making them larger and rounder, enabling them to deliver memory messages more effectively.

Mother's milk is high in choline, with the content being highest the first few days after birth. Meck thinks that choline in mother's milk is of "critical importance in memory development, the determination of adult memory capacity, and resistance to age-related memory impairments." By contrast, infant formula is far lower in choline content than breast milk, a fact that Meck thinks could impact upon the individual's future cognitive capacity.*

*Pregnant women should consult their physician before trying this.

CHOLINE AND LECITHIN

Choline and lecithin enable the body to produce acetylcholine, which transmits electrical impulses to the brain and nervous system,

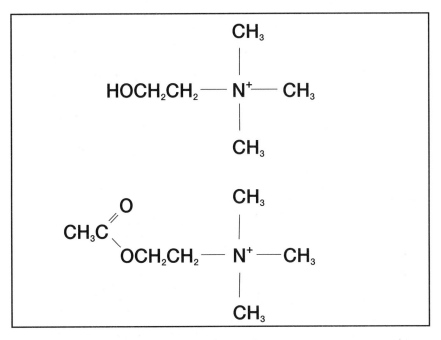

CHOLINE & ACETYLCHOLINE FORMULAS: The neurotransmitter acetyl-choline is made from choline and acetate. Lecithin is a good source of choline.

FROM *SECRETS OF LIFE EXTENSION* BY JOHN MANN, AND/OR PRESS, ©1980 . PERMISSION TO REPRINT GRANTED BY RONIN PUBLISHING, INC., BERKELEY, CA. ALL RIGHTS RESERVED.

and is essential for storing memories and for optimal mental functioning. Since choline and lecithin together are precursors for this vital neurotransmitter, they play a key role in making the brain work properly.

The brain makes acetylcholine from choline in foods such as fish and from lecithin in seed oils. Pearson and Shaw report that MIT students taking 3 grams of choline a day showed improved ability to recall a list of words. Improved memory is usually evident a few days after beginning to take choline or lecithin.

Lecithin in liquid form is a thick, viscous substance that is largely tasteless and resembles some kind of lubricant. The commercial form is found in all kinds of foods, especially candy bars like Milky Way. It is the lecithin that keeps the chocolate smooth and milky. This commercial lecithin is an emulsifier that enables fat-soluble and water-soluble substances to mix smoothly. In the body this form of lecithin emulsifies cholesterol, keeping it liquid, so that it will not harden into deposits in the arteries.

The second kind of lecithin, technically called phosphatidyl choline, is an important structural component of brain cells. It is converted by the body into choline, which is essential for acetylcholine production. This is the kind of lecithin found in health-food stores in liquid, granules, and powders. This type of lecithin nourishes the fatty sheaths covering the nerve fibers. According to Adele Davis, author of the classic *Let's Get Well,* 30 percent of the dry weight of the brain is attributed to lecithin.

The brain does manufacture acetylcholine from choline and lecithin obtained from foods we eat. But as we age, the process becomes less efficient, so that the brain produces less acetylcholine, which is then destroyed at a faster rate by free radicals. The result is diminished memory and mental functioning. Because of this decline in acetylcholine production, experts recommend supplements and eating foods rich in lecithin, such as soybeans and seed oils. Other foods high in lecithin are liver, egg yolks, peanuts, peas, beans, brewer's yeast, green leafy vegetables, cheese, cabbage, and cauliflower.

Both choline and lecithin are available in health-food stores as nutritional supplements in liquids, capsules, and other forms. Liquid lecithin can be added to scrambled eggs, soups, and stews. Both lecithin and choline can be mixed in a blender into smart drinks. Whether to use choline or lecithin or both is a matter of personal taste, since they are equally beneficial in brain boosting. Of course, lecithin offers the added benefit of emulsifying cholesterol. About 2.5 to 3 grams of choline should be taken four times a day to keep blood levels high. Lecithin, which acts like a timed-released form of choline, needs to be taken only twice daily. Somewhat more lecithin than choline can be taken, because only part of the lecithin is choline.

Both Mann and Pelton recommend taking vitamin B_5 along with choline or lecithin. Vitamin B_5 in ample amounts (usually one gram a day) is needed to convert choline to acetylcholine. Sometimes people taking choline develop a fishy body odor, which is caused by intestinal bacteria breaking down the choline. It can be eliminated by eating yogurt and drinking acidophilus milk. Alternatively, you can use lecithin instead of choline. Choline in large doses can cause diarrhea and excessive muscle tone, which may produce symptoms such as stiff neck, muscle tension, headaches, or gastric cramps. Again, lecithin doesn't have this side effect.

EGG LECITHIN

Another form of lecithin developed by Israeli researchers, called AL721, is made from egg yolk. The peculiar name was derived because it is made of seven parts neutral oils or lipids, two parts phosphatidyl choline (the form of choline found in lecithin), and one part of another chemical substance called phosphatidyl ethanolamine. However, if you look for the substance in stores, it has a commercial name, EggsACT, which highlights the egg-yolk connection.

The substance was developed to treat senility and viral diseases, including AIDS. However, it also improves memory and mental functioning. Researchers believe that AL721 makes the cell membranes in the brain more fluid. Because most of the cell's electrochemical activity begins in these membranes, these researchers believe that greater fluidity makes the cell's metabolism more stable. Other researchers believe the substance improves intelligence by providing cells with the basic materials needed for creating and repairing the membranes. Still others think that AL721 simply provides additional precursors for making acetylcholine, though they think it's an overly expensive way of providing this.

But whatever the reason that lecithin derived from egg yolks improves thinking and intelligence, what is important is that research has shown that it works. For example, Dean and Morgenthaler report in *Smart Drugs & Nutrients* that when a group of researchers gave the compound to a sample of elderly people, their cognitive abilities improved. Consumers of the product in health-food stores have reported that they were able to think better, too.

Some 2 to 10 grams per day is the suggested dose of AL721 for cognitive enhancement. Like other types of choline and lecithin, AL721 should be taken with vitamin B_5, which is needed to convert choline into acetylcholine.

AMINO ACIDS

All neurotransmitters are made from amino acids. The functioning of the brain relies greatly on the presence in the diet of important building blocks of amino acids. Often, certain foods are called "brain foods" because they contain the building blocks of the neurotransmitters. Amino acids are important to brain chemistry and emotions. Some mood disorders are caused by a deficiency or an excess of certain neurotransmitters. For example, a deficiency of some amino acids can inhibit adrenaline production, which influences the stress response. Insufficient amounts of certain amino acids can result in feeling depressed and lethargic. By increasing the intake of the correct amino acid, one will feel more energetic and in a happier mood.

Amino acids are the metabolic building blocks of all protein molecules. The body uses the amino acids to build more complex proteins. The amino acids are considered either essential or nonessential. Essential amino acids must be obtained directly, because the body cannot manufacture them. Nonessential amino acids can be manufactured in the body from essential amino acids. It doesn't mean that they are not essential for survival, but refers to whether or not they can be manufactured from amino acids available in the body.

Free-form amino acids are amino acids that have been extracted from complex proteins in vegetable products such as molasses and soybeans. Vegetarians like them because they can get the amino acids they need without having to eat meat-based products.

Amino acids come in L and D forms. The L-form amino acids can be used directly by the body as proteins, and are easily absorbed and used. The body must convert D-form amino acids before they can be absorbed and used. Sale of the D form is usually prohibited by the FDA. Robert Erdmann, author of *The Amino Revolution*, advised that consumers check to insure that powdered amino-acid supplements specify the quantity of free-form amino acids. If the label says only "amino acid," it is probably mostly cheap protein-powder filler, with very little of any particular amino acid.

It is important to take amino acids with cofactors, which are usually vitamins, minerals, or other nutrients that help the amino acids to be metabolized. Erdmann recommends taking amino acids in combination rather than one amino-acid supplement by itself, because the working of amino acids involve complex metabolic pathways in which the cofactors and related amino acids are required.

PHENYLALANINE

The amino acid most widely considered a brain booster and a common ingredient in smart drinks is phenylalanine. It is an essential amino acid, available from natural sources such as beef, chicken, fish, soybeans, eggs, cottage cheese, and milk. It is digested and absorbed in the liver, where some amount of it is used to regulate blood sugar through insulin. Phenylalanine also contributes to the production of protein fiber in the cells.

Phenylalanine is a building block in the metabolic chain reaction that creates the neurotransmitters called catecholamines, including norepinephrine and dopamine, which cause mental arousal, alertness, and elevated moods. The best known catecholamines are norepinephrine and adrenaline, which create the fight–flight response to stress and increase alertness, stamina, and strength. Production of adrenaline and noradrenaline are stimulated by stress. Unrelenting stress uses up the available noradrenaline. About the process, Durk Pearson says, "Eventually you're totally drained, not just physically, but mentally, too." According to Pearson, phenylalanine is converted into noradrenaline. Unlike coffee, which uses up noradrenaline and, after a stressful five to ten cup of coffee day, can leave one feeling jittery and irritable, phenylalanine can help one function at peak levels and able to handle stress, danger, and excitement.

BRAIN DRAIN

"Brain drain" is a common syndrome in our fast-paced culture. If you've got any doubt, just look at how much coffee we consume. Coffee is one of the largest commodities traded in the world, second only to petroleum. The caffeine in coffee works in part to keep us alert and active by activating the noradrenaline system. Noradrenaline is a neurotransmitter and the brain's version of adrenaline. When under stress, "you're using up noradrenaline much faster than you can make it," explained Durk Pearson, author of *Life Extension*. "Eventually, you're totally drained, not just physically, but mentally too." But like a car running out of gas, coffee does nothing to replenish the noradrenaline it uses up. By the end of a stressful four or five cup day, the jitteriness and irritability you feel are signs that you're literally running on empty, at least with regard to noradrenaline.

When your noradrenaline system is functioning at peak level, your awareness is heightened, and you're primed to handle heavy stress, danger, or excitement. The neurons that produce noradrenaline originate primarily in a region of the brain known as the locus cœruleus. Although few in number, their influence is profound, since they branch out to nearly every part of the brain and spinal cord.

The amino-acid phenylalanine can help to keep the noradrenaline stores full, so you avoid the "running on empty" syndrome—the let-down you get from drinking coffee.

Intelli-Scope
The Newsletter of the Designer Foods™ Network

According to Erdmann, phenylalanine can alleviate depression and has been found to improve learning potential. Erdmann cautions not to use MAO (Monoamine Oxidase) inhibitors and amino acids at the same time. He also cautions people who are taking L-phenylalanine to do so under guidance of a doctor or a nutritionist, and to have blood pressure monitored regularly. Excessive consumption of L-phenylalanine may make some people overstimulated and irritable, and may cause insomnia, especially when taken in the late afternoon or evening. Reducing the amount consumed usually eliminates this reaction. Insomnia can be avoided by taking it only once a day in the mornings. Pearson and Shaw caution that no more than 2.4 grams of supplemental phenylalanine per day should be taken.

Andrew Weil, author of *Natural Health, Natural Medicine,* on the other hand, does not recommend taking amino acids as nutritional supplements. He does note, however, that phenylalanine can be helpful in some cases of depression, and useful for people with chronic pain.

Andrew Weil suggests using a blend of the D and L form of phenylalanine, also known as DL-phenylalanine or DLPA, for relief of depression or for increased energy. His formula involves taking 1,000 to 1,500 mg. of DLPA in the morning on an empty stomach, and again later in the day with 100 mg. of vitamin B_6, 500 mg. of vitamin C, and a piece of fruit or a glass of fruit juice. He reports that people using this formula experience mental arousal, increased energy level, and elevated mood.

Andrew Weil recommends that people with high blood pressure start with lower doses, of 100 mg. of DLPA, and raise the doses gradually over a few weeks as they monitor blood pressure. Pearson and Shaw caution that phenylalanine should not be used by persons with the genetic metabolic disorder PKU, psychosis, anyone taking MAO-inhibitor drugs, pigmented malignant melanoma cancer, or Wilson's disease. They warn that it should not be given to children and recommend that pregnant or lactating women consult a physician before using phenylalanine.

METABOLIC PATHWAYS

Metabolic pathways are the body's biochemical assembly
lines, which take the raw materials, such as newly eaten
amino acids, and manufacture finished products to help the
body to live. Making sure that the metabolic pathways work
at peak performance means ensuring that your body has all
the raw materials that it needs: vitamins, minerals, and,
most important of all, amino acids.

Robert Erdmann
The Amino Revolution

The amino acids tyrosine and methionine are important amino acids
used in conjunction with DLPA. Tyrosine is part of the chemical
pathway in the creation of adrenaline and noradrenaline. Methionine is
a sulfur-based amino acid. Mineral sulfur protects cells from air-borne
pollutants like smoke and auto exhaust, and transports selenium and
zinc around the body. Sulfur slows down the aging process and aids in
protein production. Methionine is found in dairy products, eggs, and
meat, but there is very little in vegetables. Vegetarians can benefit from
methionine supplements. Methionine is a chelator. It locates heavy
metals, such as lead, cadmium, and mercury, grabs onto them, and
eliminates them from the body.

ENERGY PICK-ME-UP

To combat lethargy, confusion, inability to concentrate,
and the "blahs," Erdmann recommends in *The Amino
Revolution* that this blend be taken three times a day:
• Amino acid:
  glutamine
• Cofactors:
  folic acid
  vitamin B_6
  vitamin C

GLUTAMINE

Glutamic acid or glutamine is another free-form amino acid widely used to maintain good brain functioning. Glutamine is a brain fuel that improves clarity of thinking, mental alertness, and mood. It produces the brain chemical glutamic acid, used in neutralizing ammonia metabolic waste. It also produces a neurotransmitter called gamma amino butyric acid, or GABA, which has a soothing, calming effect. Glutamic acid is used in treating epilepsy and mental retardation. Often, people use it simply as a pick-me-up.

Ammonia is a by-product of the brain metabolism when proteins are broken down. When ammonia levels get too high in the brain, one can get irritable, and experience nausea and vomiting. Eventually, one experiences tremors and hallucinations. If the condition is not alleviated, it will lead to death. The urea cycle is the metabolic pathway that converts ammonia to urea to be excreted in urine. The process begins when glutamic acid reacts with ammonia to produce glutamine. When there is a deficiency of glutamic acid, ammonia levels in the brain will increase. Even a small rise of ammonia in the brain causes fatigue, confusion, inability to concentrate, and mood swings.

The blood-brain barrier is a membrane that protects the brain cells from poisons carried in the blood. Some nutrients can cross the barrier, and others can not. Glutamic acid does not cross the blood-brain barrier; so taking glutamic acid can be futile. It doesn't reach its target in the brain, where most of the metabolism takes place, and where ammonia waste accumulates. Glutamine can cross the blood-brain barrier, however. Consequently, people usually take glutamine as a supplement. Once in the brain, glutamine is converted into glutamic acid, which goes to work detoxifying ammonia. Glutamine is also used by cells like glucose for metabolic energy.

Erdmann reports that students taking glutamine supplements find it easier to concentrate on homework and to work late into the night without fatigue. He says that taking glutamine is "almost like plugging your brain into a free fuel source." Stimulants like caffeine create alertness, but do not fuel metabolism. Glutamine actually is itself a fuel creating energy in the brain. People using glutamine report feeling livelier. Erdmann reports that students taking glutamine before tests feel more clearheaded, alert, and confident during exams.

ARGININE

Arginine is an amino acid that is converted in the body to spermine, which is found in semen, blood tissue, and brain cells. Low levels of spermine are associated with senility and memory loss. The manufacture of spermine from arginine is complicated and involves several cofactors. Here's how the metabolic pathway works.

An enzyme activated by manganese reacts with arginine to produce ornithine, another amino acid, which then reacts with vitamin B_6 to produce putrescine. Simultaneously, magnesium reacts with methionine, another amino acid, to produce activated methionine, which then converts putrescine to spermidine and then to spermine. This complicated process can be facilitated by taking supplements of the various amino acids and cofactors utilized in the process.

MEMORY-ENHANCING FORMULA

Erdmann suggests taking the following blend of nutrients once or twice a day between meals.

- Amino acids:
  methionine
  arginine
  ornithine
- Cofactors:
  vitamin B_6
  vitamin C
  manganese
  magnesium

Arginine can aggravate herpes symptoms. People with a history of herpes should consult a doctor or nutritionist before using it as a supplement.

TRYPTOPHAN

Another amino acid that is important in brain functioning is tryptophan. It is the metabolic precursor of serotonin, a very important neurotransmitter. In the late 1980s and early 1990s, tryptophan was used widely to relieve anxiety and enhance sleep. It was readily available in health-food stores.

After thirty-eight people who used tryptophan died, and hundreds developed a blood disorder attributed to L-tryptophan, the FDA banned its sale in the early 1990s in the United States. Questions arose about whether the deaths were a result of one contaminated batch or due to something inherent in the chemical itself. Andrew Weil does not recommend using L-tryptophan until the causes of the problems are clearly established.

SELENIUM

Selenium is a trace element that is essential for health and optimal mental functioning. It detoxifies heavy metals, most notably lead, mercury, arsenic, and cadmium, which are toxic and upset brain chemistry. Metals enter the body through the foods we eat, the air we breathe, and the water we drink. Heavy-metal poisoning is increasing because of pollutants in the environment. Analysis of human hair taken from people living today and from people who died 1,600 years ago shows that traces of metal in hair are now up to a thousand times greater.

Even a tiny amount of metals like lead or mercury can interfere with thinking and memory by disturbing brain chemistry. Removing toxic metals can put our mental functioning back on track. A small amount of lead in the body will cause learning disorders, mental retardation, and lower I.Q. scores in children. Lead can accumulate in the tissues until it reaches lethal levels, and so is particularly dangerous. Ceramic glazes often contain lead to create brilliant colors, but this renders the dishes poisonous. Paints in old buildings often contain high lead content. Every year there are several cases of ghetto children being poisoned by eating paint chips. Research shows that selenium removes lead from the body. When lead is removed, mental functioning can be restored and I.Q. increased.

Mercury is another metal that can damage the brain. Like lead, it accumulates in the tissues, can interfere with brain functioning, and may even cause premature senility. Some of the first signs of poisoning include being tired, having headaches, and forgetting things. Later, one might experience difficulties with speech, hearing, and remembering things. Also, there may be problems concentrating.

Selenium can clear up the problems caused by exposure to toxic metals. For example, selenium combines with methyl mercury to make it soluble for excretion. The process works a little like a vacuum cleaner cleaning a house. The selenium comes in, sucks up the toxic metals, then throws them away. So to speak, selenium cleans up the brain like cleaning up a house.

Selenium is a powerful antioxidant and deactivates free radicals. Working in conjunction with the antioxidant glutathione peroxidase, an antioxidant enzyme, it triggers conversion of lipid peroxides into harmless hydroxy acids, and thereby protects cell membranes and tissues from destruction by free radicals. Selenium has a synergistic effect when taken with vitamin E. Both are powerful antioxidants that neutralize free radicals, and selenium makes vitamin E more effective.

Brewer's yeast, whole-grain breads and cereals, wheat germ, bran, and barley are high in selenium, if grown on selenium-rich soil. Tuna, herring, and shellfish, organ meats like liver and kidneys, and dairy products like eggs are rich in selenium.

Selenium has benefits beyond protecting the brain from heavy metals. Pelton calls it "a nutritional superstar" because of its anticancer effects, its benefits to the immune system, and its protection against disease of the heart and circulatory system. We need selenium to resist disease. Taking selenium with vitamin E can increase antibodies thirtyfold.

Selenium is toxic in high doses, even though it is essential for health. There is considerable debate about the optimal dose. Pelton's review suggests daily supplements of 100 to 300 micrograms a day. Mann reports positive results with much higher doses, up to 3,000 micrograms a day. Considering the potential for taking too much, it is probably a good idea to be conservative and to take high doses only after consulting a physician. Pelton argues persuasively for the superiority of organic selenium, which is higher in nutritional value and better absorbed by the body.

FATS AND OILS

The brain cells are 60 percent fat, which is a much higher percentage than in other parts of the body. It is ironic that people constantly try to cut fats out of their diets, because having enough fats is essential for developing and maintaining a well-functioning brain.

There are two essential fatty acids, alpha-linolenic acid, called Omega-3, and linoleic acid, called Omega-6. They are referred to as "essential," because the body manufactures all the other fats it needs from these two essentials.

The fat we are least likely to get in our diet is the alpha-linolenic or Omega-3, which is the one we need the most. A deficiency of essential fatty acids is one of the major causes of chronic degenerative diseases, such as cancer, heart disease, high blood pressure, and strokes. And without these essential fatty acids, there is a decline in brain functioning, too.

Although we probably get a lot of fat in our diets, it's usually the wrong kind, from beef and hydrogenated oils. Partially hydrogenated fats and oils contain toxic fats that can harm the brain. The hydrogenation process forces hydrogen gas into the fat molecules and alters their structure, making the oil dangerous to health and mental functioning. Once the hydrogenated fat gets into the cell walls, it interferes with the transfer of nutrients through the wall. The result is toxic buildup and malnourished cells. Hydrogenated fat is also called saturated oil, because the molecular chains are occupied or saturated with hydrogen atoms. It is widely used in margarine, vegetable shortenings, shortening oil, and processed salad dressings because of its resistance to rancidity. Most nutritionists recommend avoiding hydrogenated fats and using fresh oils made from seeds. When you consider that fat is the building material of brain cells, it makes sense to use natural oils and avoid those altered by hydrogenation.

However, the fact that fats are natural and unprocessed still doesn't mean they are good for you. Unprocessed oils come in three forms: saturated, polyunsaturated, and monounsaturated. Saturated fats have been implicated in cholesterol buildup, heart disease, cancer, and other serious illnesses. Saturated oils are easy to recognize because they become hard and opaque in the cold. Animal fats are saturated. They look like hard, white veins in meats.

ANDREW WEIL'S FAT RECOMMENDATIONS

- Avoid fats at either extreme of the saturated–unsaturated spectrum.
- Do not eat cookies, crackers, breads, or pastries containing partially hydrogenated anything.
- Minimize intake of polyunsaturated oils and products made from them.
- Don't heat polyunsaturated oils. Use them only in salads and other cold foods.
- Substitute monounsaturated fats for polyunsaturated fats.
- Buy oils in small quantities, not giant size.
- Always refrigerate oils after opening.
- Never reuse an oil that has been heated to high temperatures. Throw it out.
- Never heat an oil to the point of smoking. Smoke from overheated oil is highly carcinogenic. It is dangerous to breathe the vapors.
- Always smell oils before using them, and discard if there is any hint of rancidity.
- Never eat anything deep-fried in fast-food restaurants.

Andrew Weil
Natural Health, Natural Medicine

Polyunsaturated fats, which are used in many salad dressings, stay transparent and free-flowing under refrigeration. But polyunsaturated fats have dangers of their own that are not widely known. They are particularly prone to oxidation, especially when heated and left exposed to air. We definitely want to keep oxidized cells out of our bodies, because they create free radicals that destroy nerve and vital organ cells, which leads to mental decline, accelerated aging, and cancer. If a polyunsaturated oil smells rancid, don't eat it. Unfortunately, most deep-fried fast foods, like French fries, are cooked in rancid oils. Think about it. They are heated up over and over, and left sometimes for days exposed to air. In the middle between saturated and polyunsaturated are monounsaturated fats. Olive, canola, and peanut oils are monounsaturated.

Omega-3 provides a fluid and the needed energy to help move the impulses carrying messages from one brain cell to another. By facilitation of the transmission of messages, it enables us to think, store, and retrieve memories. It is necessary for developing embryos, too. Researchers have found from animal studies that babies will have irreversible learning disabilities when the mother is deficient in Omega-3 fats. It is also needed for healthy eye retinas, operation of synapses, and handling stress.

Flaxseed, or linseed, as it is also known, pumpkin, wheat germ, canola, soybean, and walnut oils are good sources of unsaturated oils that provide essential fatty acids. They should always be kept refrigerated and used only if fresh, because Omega-3 fat is destroyed by heat, light, and exposure to oxygen. Salmon, mackerel, trout, sardines, tuna, and eel are good sources of Omega-3. In fact, fish oil in general is an excellent source of Omega-3 fats. Primrose oil is a good source of Omega-6 fats.

ROYAL JELLY

Royal jelly is a fascinating and mysterious food manufactured by bees. It is a thick, milky substance made from pollen and honey, and secreted from the pharyngeal glands of young nurse bees between their sixth and

ANDREW WEIL COMMENTS ON OILS

Oils are listed from most unsaturated to most saturated. The value in the parentheses indicates the amount of monounsaturated fats.

Safflower (12%): Too unsaturated; avoid it.

Sunflower, corn, sesame (11%): Too high in unsaturated fat; use moderately and do not heat.

Sesame, roasted (dark): A highly flavored seasoning used in Oriental dishes. Add small amounts to soup and stir-fries after cooking. Use in salad dressings and marinades.

Nut oils (walnut, hazelnut): Expensive, flavorful, polyunsaturated. Use moderately in salads, marinades, and cold dishes.

Soy (24%): Cheap, similar to corn in composition, mostly polyunsaturated. Use moderately, if at all, and do not heat.

Cottonseed (19%): Too high in saturated fat, too low in monounsaturated fat. Also, because cotton is not classed as a food crop, the oil may contain more pesticide residues than other oils. Avoid it.

Peanut (49%): Has a good percentage of monounsaturated fat, but has more saturated fat than canola oil, and more polyunsaturated fat than olive oil. Use it moderately.

Avocado: Mostly monounsaturated, but unflavored and expensive.

Olive (77%): Provides more monounsaturated fat than any other oil. Buy only extra virgin or virgin oil, and use in both hot and cold dishes.

ANDREW WEIL COMMENTS ON OILS (*continued*)

Canola: Is substantially monounsaturated, and has less saturated fat than any other oil (less than half of olive). Use it as a general-purpose, unflavored oil.

Palm (39%) palm kernel, coconut: Too high in saturated fat; avoid them altogether.

Cocoa butter: The fat in chocolate appears hard at room temperature but may not pose as much cardiovascular risk as other saturated fats. (The body may change one of its saturated fatty acids into a monounsaturated one.) Best eaten in moderation but can be applied liberally to the skin to soothe rough, dry areas.

Vegetable shortening (Crisco) (43%): A mixture of saturated and unsaturated fats, but the oils have been deformed by chemical processing. Avoid it.

Margarine (48%): Ditto.

Chicken fat (47%), lard (47%), beef fat (44%): Too saturated. Avoid them entirely, or minimize consumption. Unlike vegetable fats, they contain cholesterol.

Butterfat (30%): The most saturated of all animal fats, and contains the most cholesterol (more than twice that of beef fat). Try to minimize consumption of butter, cream, ice cream, and whole-milk products. Read labels for the percentage of fat in these products.

Andrew Weil
Natural Health, Natural Medicine

twelfth days of life. Royal jelly is a food given to all the female larvae for the first three days after hatching. Here is the incredible thing. On day four most of the bees are switched to a diet of honey and pollen. Only the special larva selected to become the queen continues to be fed royal jelly throughout her entire life. Apiculturalists have found that the only difference between the queen and the other females is her diet of royal jelly. The queen bee is extremely fertile, and lays more than 2,000 eggs a day, which is over twice her body weight. Whereas the other bees live about three months, the queen lives four to five years.

Royal jelly, which is a natural and unprocessed food, is one of the world's richest natural sources of pantothenic acid (vitamin B_5), sometimes called the anti-stress vitamin. It is also rich in B_1, B_2, B_3, B_6, B_{12}, biotin, folic acid, and the vitamin-B-like substance inositol. It is a natural source of acetylcholine, and contains vitamins A, C, D, and E. If this isn't impressive enough, it also contains the minerals: phosphorus, which protects from stress and improves mental functioning, calcium, potassium, sulfur, iron, manganese, nickel, cobalt, silicon, chromium, gold, bismuth, and trace minerals. Royal jelly contains eighteen of the amino acids, including glutamic acid and phenylalanine. Fatty acids, enzymes, and the hormone testosterone, which is needed by both men and women, are found in royal jelly. Plus 4 percent of royal jelly has defied laboratory analysis. All of this is in a natural food. Wow, those amazing little bees!

If you've read this far in this book, you'll recognize that royal jelly contains many brain-boosting substances. The acetylcholine is an important neurotransmitter. Vitamins A, B_1, B_2, B_3, B_5, B_6, B_{12}, C, and E are antioxidants that destroy free radicals and, thereby, help preserve brain cells. Amino acids and fatty acids are important building blocks of brain cells. So it is not too surprising that royal jelly rejuvenates and improves mental alertness and concentration. It also is a powerful energy source. Honey is a very accessible natural sugar that is easily converted into glucose, the body's energy fuel. It's probably safe to say that if one were going to add only one brain food to the diet, it should be royal jelly for the maximum benefit.

A Russian study of people who lived to be a hundred years old revealed that many of them had been beekeepers. They discovered that all the centenarians, without exception, consumed honey as one of their principal foods. Dr. Ricardo Galleazzi Lisi, the physician for Pope Pius XII, publicly stated that he attributed the Pope's recovery from a long, weakening illness to his taking royal jelly. The president of Chile said that he believed that eating royal jelly helped him develop the vigor he needed to do his job. He was eighty years old at the time. Several members of the Royal family have publicly endorsed royal jelly, including Prince Phillip, Princess Anne, and Princess Margaret. It is reported that Princess Diana took royal jelly during her pregnancy. (Nonetheless, pregnant and nursing women should consult their personal physician before using royal jelly.)

Another amazing property of royal jelly is its antibacterial, antiviral, and antifungicidal activity. It is well-known that honey needs no preservatives because it resists spoiling. The reason for this is propolis, another amazing substance manufactured by bees. Propolis is a sticky material made up of wax, resin, balsam, oil, and pollen collected by bees from the buds of trees and tree bark. Crude honey from natural hives contains bits of propolis, which keeps it sterile. The ancient Assyrians and Egyptians used honey's antiseptic and embalming properties when they buried their dead in honey and beeswax. Propolis and honey have been used by Soviet surgeons, who feed it to their patients prior to surgery as a precaution to reduce infection. It has been used to heal wounds and treat skin diseases. Royal jelly inevitably contains a little propolis and honey.

Royal jelly is delicate, and loses its activation when exposed to air, room temperature, and sunlight. But when mixed with honey it is more stable. It is available in sealed capsules, frozen, freeze-dried, and mixed in honey. Irene Stein, author of *Royal Jelly: The New Guide to Nature's Richest Health Food*, recommends against the freeze-dried form, because she says that the process alters its chemical structure. Pure royal jelly can be purchased in some herb stores, such as Lhasa Karnac in Berkeley, in two-ounce jars. This most-potent form is very unstable, and should always be kept refrigerated. The recommended daily serving is about 1/3 teaspoon, or a large drop. If you try it this way, be prepared, because the taste is definitely strange, and gives the impression that you are eating bee milk. We find it is more palatable to mix the pure royal jelly with a teaspoon of honey.

Stein says that the best royal jelly comes from China. If you visit Chinatown, you can find inexpensive boxes of phials of royal jelly mixed with ginseng in grocery stores. Drinking one of these provides a fast-acting pick-me-up. Stein recommends taking 150 mg. a day in capsules or mixed with honey. Premier One, which packages royal jelly for health stores, recommends 600 mg. a day. When taken with honey, it can be spread on bread for a wonderful breakfast food. But royal jelly should never be mixed with hot liquids, since this destroys the beneficial properties. And you should not drink hot liquids right after taking royal jelly. Increased energy is noticed very quickly. However, it must be taken regularly for several weeks before most people notice improved mental functioning and concentration.

SMART DRINKS

Smart drinks are nutrient cocktails that are often served at parties and raves by smart bars as an alternative to alcohol. They are made from fast-dissolving mixtures of vitamins, minerals, and amino acids. There are two general categories of smart drinks: pick-me-ups, which are claimed to increase energy and stamina; and mental tonics, which are claimed to improve thinking and memory. Best-known are those based on Durk Pearson and Sandy Shaw's formulas, Blast™ (with caffeine) and Rise and Shine™ (without caffeine), which are energizers, and Memory Fuel™, which is a brain food. Earth Girl's Get Smart Think Drinks™ include Energy Elicksure™ and Psuper Psonic Psyber Tonic™. Although the exact formulas differ in the amounts of each ingredient, they all contain a long list of vitamins and minerals. The key ingredient in the energy drinks is phenylalanine, which activates noradrenaline, which is the brain's version of adrenaline and an essential neurotransmitter, whereas choline is the key ingredient in the brain-food drinks. Choline is converted in the brain into acetylcholine, a neurotransmitter

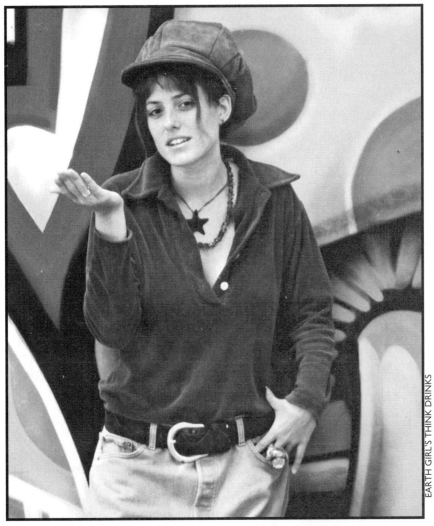

EARTH GIRL'S THINK DRINKS

Earth Girl, creator of "Get Smart Think Drinks," and a catalyst in the smart drinks phenomenon.

critical for proper memory functioning. Earth Girl's Psuper Psonic Psyber Tonic also contains phenylalanine and *Ginkgo biloba*, an herb with cognitive-enhancing qualities.

Smart drinks are made by mixing a well-rounded tablespoon of the product in four to eight ounces of ice-cold water or fruit juice, and serving it over ice. They have a tangy citrus flavor, and make a perfect breakfast drink. Best results are claimed to result when it is drunk immediately after awakening, on an empty stomach, or an hour before a meal, or at snack time to help satisfy hunger. All smart drinks products carry lengthy cautionary statements that should be read and followed. Smart drinks should never be given to children, or to pregnant or lactating women. Because smart drinks usually contain amino acids, they are not advised for people taking MAO inhibitors.

The Pearson and Shaw products are easier to find, and can be purchased by fax or phone from Smart Products in San Francisco. But Earth Girl's drinks are more fun. For example, the label of Psuper Psonic Psyber Tonic reads: "A Cosmadelicious Think Drink™ Hyper-fruitful lemon-cherry memory-friendly neuro-nectar™ Lets you be the star that you are! Earth Girl's Mission: "CONGRATULATIONS EARTHLINKS and Welcome to the Wonderful World of NOW. It's the only time we have—so why waste it? It's all about you! Maximize. Utilize. Visualize. Realize that beauty lies in your potential-wise existence; Let Go of your Resistance. WAKE UP AND LOVE. Increase your Sensitivity. Expand all Possibilities. Exercise the Ability to improve your Reality. LIGHT UP AND LIVE. You are invited to stop brain and body pollution. Join the intelligence revolution. Personal evolution is the global solution. START NOW! Your participation in this mission is essential! Love attracts Love" (signed) Earth Girl. Adding to the fun is the "psecret psurprise" inside. Each jar contains a small trinket like the old Cracker Jacks boxes did.

Literature distributed to bar wholesalers and distributors of the Pearson and Shaw products cautions against the use of the word "smart." It says: "The FDA currently objects to the use of the word 'smart' in conjunction with vitamin and amino-acid formulations; so the popular catchphrases "Smart Bar' and 'Smart Drink' cannot be used except within the context of a statement such as 'Smart Bars Provide an Intelligent Alternative to Alcohol.' Do not state or imply that these drinks make one smarter, improve intelligence, or can be used in the treatment of any illness or injury. No such claim is made or implied by the manufacturer or its distributors."

VITAMIN AND MINERAL COCKTAILS

Virtually all experts on health, including the Surgeon General, the Secretary of Health and Human Services, and our grandmothers, have given the same advice: Eat more fruits and vegetables. We've all heard this advice, but few of us heed it. How much of our diet should be fruits and vegetables is hotly debated. In fact, increasingly the evidence points to the importance of eating fruits and vegetables raw. When cooked they lose a lot of their nutrients. Processed and packaged foods have the additional problems of preservatives. But eaten raw, the nutrients in fruits and vegetables are actually consumed "alive" and unchanged. There's no heating and processing to sap nutrients, no additives to pose unknown health risks. Reading through the many vitamins, minerals, and fats described in this book that promote mental functioning, we see that many are found in high quantities in fruits and vegetables. And if you're like a lot of people, when you read the list of foods high in beta-carotene, for example, you shake your head and think, "Yea, I should eat more carrots and spinach."

Calbom and Keane, in *Juicing for Life,* say that each person should eat at least two bowls of raw food every day, but very few Americans do so. In fact, most Americans eat only one to three salads each week! And then the salad is often covered with a heavy fat-rich dressing. Our busy lifestyles are part of the problem. We just don't have time. We often skip breakfast, grab fast food for lunch, and microwave a frozen meal for dinner. Juicing is a fast, inexpensive solution to making a habit of consuming the large quantities of fruits and vegetables needed for optimal health, good mental functioning, and longevity.

The key to juicing is to buy a juicer that you will use. Virtually any fruit or vegetable is a good candidate for the juicer, especially when blended with others. When you take supplements, especially in high doses, you must be fairly knowledgeable about what you need to make up a balanced diet. Often you have to take other nutrients to balance your supplements. It can be very complicated and confusing. And sometimes, if you're not careful, you can create deficiencies by taking too much of one nutrient. This is particularly true with the B vitamins, which the body needs in certain ratios.

VEGGIE COCKTAIL FOR PREVENTING ALZHEIMER'S

handful of wheatgrass	1/2 handful of parsley
handful of watercress	4 carrots, green removed
3 stalks celery	1/2 cup chopped fennel
1/2 apple, seeded	

Bunch up wheatgrass, parsley, and watercress, and push through juice hopper with carrots, celery, fennel, and apple. Drink.

Cherie Calbom & Maureen Keane
Juicing for Life

With juices you don't have this problem. The remarkable thing about natural foods, especially raw foods, is that they usually contain several vitamins, minerals, and enzymes in the right balance. And they work together synergistically. You don't have to become a junior chemist concocting combinations of pills. Instead, you can just juice up a bunch of vegetables into a wonderful vitamin and mineral cocktail, and drink your way to clearer thinking and longer life.

BRAIN-BOOSTER SNACKS

Blend until smooth a freshly juiced apple and a cup of cashew nuts in a food processor. Chill the mixture until it thickens. Spread on whole-wheat crackers and serve.

Eat seeds and nut butters, which are rich in Omega-3 fats. The fats stimulate the release of neurotransmitters that can help you think better and remember more.

Calbom and Keane report evidence that autopsies of Alzheimer's victims show large deposits of aluminum and silicon in their brains. They recommend that all sources of aluminum be removed from daily

SEBASTIAN'S GET-SMART PESTO

4 bunches of basil	1/2 cup canola or olive oil
bunch of parsley	1/2 cup pine nuts
bunch of spinach	1/2 cup chopped walnuts
1 head fresh garlic	1 cup ground Parmesan cheese
food processor	small frying pan

Lightly toast the nuts in a small amount of oil until golden and set aside. Peel garlic and put it in food processor. Add oil. Purée garlic and oil. Switch food-processor setting to chop. Add basil, parsley, and spinach to the puréed garlic and oil in food processor, and chop. Pour contents of food processor into a large bowl, add cheese and nuts, and mix by hand.

The very thick pesto mix can be spread on whole-grain crackers and eaten as an hors d'oeuvre. As a spread, the garlic in the pesto can be a little hot and nippy. Eat one or two teaspoons. If too hot, place pesto to be used in microwave, and cook for thirty seconds. Test for nippiness again, and repeat cooking if still too hot.

For traditional pesto, prepare rotelle noodles or spaghetti noodles al dente (a little chewy). Drain and put into a large bowl. Add 2 to 3 three heaping tablespoons of pesto for each cup of cooked noodles and mix. The hot noodles will cook the garlic and eliminate its nippiness.

Leftover pesto can be divided into two- to four-person servings, placed in small plastic containers, and frozen for future use. Frozen pesto should be removed from freezer about half an hour before being added to hot noodles.

Spinach, parsley, and basil are sources of beta-carotene, vitamin-B complex, and vitamin C, which are all antioxidants. Since the greens are not cooked, except for the heat of the noodles, virtually all their nutrients are present. Garlic has substantial levels of selenium, another antioxidant. Canola and olive oil are both monounsaturated oils, which are good sources of Omega-3 fats; yet they are reasonably resistant to oxidation. The nuts are a good source of amino acids, lecithin and Omega-3 fats. Finally, the cheese, although it is high in animal fats, is a good source of amino acids.

use. Some drinking water contains aluminum. Bottled water can be substituted. Cook in stainless-steel cookware, and avoid aluminum pots and pans. Many over-the-counter medicines and cosmetics are high in aluminum, and should be avoided; these include buffered aspirin, some toothpastes, antiperspirants, diarrhea medicines, dandruff shampoos, and makeup. Read the label for aluminum content. They recommend avoiding products in aluminum containers, such as beers and colas. Additionally, they suggest avoiding processed cheese, because it usually contains aluminum. Calbom and Keane offer several juice recipes that are high in the mineral and antioxidants that they say are good for helping to prevent Alzheimer's disease.

Overall, we think you will have noticed in this chapter that "eating smart" does not restrict you to a boring diet. In fact, if you're anything like most Americans, the recommendations here should inspire you to consume a much more varied and cosmopolitan menu of healthy foods.

11

HERBAL SMART FOODS

Besides smart nutrients, vitamins, minerals, and drugs, certain herbs and spices can boost brain power. Herbs are plants used for nutrition or for therapeutic purposes, whereas spices are aromatic vegetable substances used to add flavor to foods and beverages or to prevent food from spoiling.

DISTINGUISHING BETWEEN HERBS AND SPICES

Whether a plant is called an herb or a spice depends on how it is used rather than what it is. Plants we normally think of as herbs can be considered spices when used for flavoring or preservative purposes. For example, we think of salt as a spice when we use it to flavor food, even though it is a mineral. So the distinction between herb and spice can be almost casual. In the following discussion, *herb* will be used to refer to the plants used for food, healing, or mental improvement. *Spices* will refer to substances used to improve taste or to make nutrients last longer. In *Life Extension*, Pearson and Shaw discuss the antioxidant effect of spices in preserving food; they work much like synthetic antioxidants, such as BHT and BHA. Cloves, oregano, sage, rosemary, and vanilla are examples. Other spices with antioxidizing powers include frankincense and myrrh, which have been used for thousands of years as a preservative, as cited in the Bible.

DISTINGUISHING HERBS FROM NUTRIENTS AND DRUGS

We've already seen that distinctions can be fuzzy in this world of smart drugs and nutrients. Sometimes one may use an herb because it tastes good; sometimes as a medication to feel better or prevent a disease; at yet other times for both purposes. For example, an herb or blend of herbs can be made into a tea to be a refreshing beverage as well as a therapeutic tonic. Herbs differ from vegetables served as a food dish in that herbs are usually chopped up, powdered, added to food, brewed into a tea, or made into a poultice to be applied to the body.

The distinction between drugs and herbs is that herbs occur in nature and have a general therapeutic effect on the body as a whole. Herbs usually act in a soothing, gentle way that promotes a better environment for the body to heal itself. By contrast, drugs are created by refining or purifying a naturally occurring substance to create a concentration of the substance and used for a specific healing or other purpose. The effects of drugs are usually stronger, in some cases, even harsh.

In the West, medical use of herbs was usurped from its medicinal role by the medical establishment's propensity for more powerful chemical drugs. It echoes Dupont's famous line: "Better living through chemistry." In *Mind Foods and Smart Pills*, Pelton notes that enterprising chemists in the eighteenth and nineteenth centuries, operating on the theory that a particular chemical substance is needed to counteract a particular disease believed to have a single cause, sought to extract the essential ingredient in herbal substances to create standardized drugs. As a result, Westerners tend to look askance at herbal medicines, since such natural plant therapies treat the whole body with the goal of bringing the body into alignment and balance. The philosophy underlying herbal treatment is that herbs energize and stimulate the body, and help the immune system function better to enable the body to heal and stay in good health. This holistic approach is traditional in other cultures, like those found in Latin America and Asia. In the West, use of herbs has generally been limited to spicing foods to perk up the flavor.

WHAT HERBS DO

There's a lot of controversy about herbal brain boosters. Some medical experts believe herbs are not particularly useful and accuse herbalists of exaggerating their effects. With few exceptions most herbal preparations are harmless. So the real question for most herbal treatments is efficacy: Does it actually have the intended effect?

It can be difficult to tell exactly what different herbs do, since traditionally their active substances have not been analyzed and identified precisely. The strength and amount of the active ingredients can differ widely, depending on where an herb is grown. Where the soil conditions and climate are more favorable, an herb can contain more and stronger amounts of particular ingredients, for example. The time of harvest can be another factor in an herb's potency. How the herb is prepared and the active ingredients extracted are important in preserving the desired activity of the plant.

Herbology has always been an inexact science. Knowledge about what herbs do has been developed and passed on by tribal and folk practices. Little scientific research has been done. Of course, we in the West tend to discount anything that hasn't been established by the scientific method.

Often combinations of herbs are used to make each more effective. For example, an herb may be added to a blend because it makes the primary herb in the blend more effective or increases the rate at which it is absorbed into the body or transported through the blood. According to Dr. Mowrey, the author of *The Scientific Validation of Herbal Medicine*, it is actually better to combine herbs than to use them separately, because this powerful blending effect enhances what the primary herb or herbs in the combo do.

Loose herbs are often of little effect because the active ingredients in the plants deteriorate when exposed to air, light, and moisture. Even encapsulated powders tend to have reduced potency, because powdering of herbs accelerates oxidation.

Dr. Andrew Weil advises that the best way to get the maximum potency is from tinctures and freeze-dried extracts. Tinctures are liquid

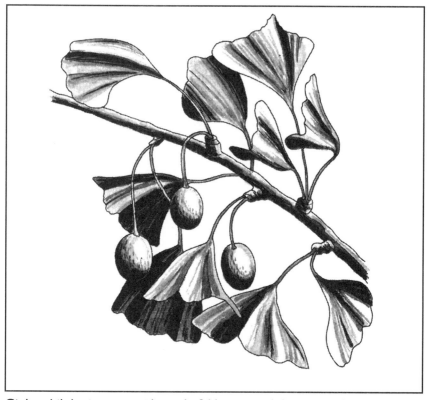

Ginkgo biloba *is a tree with a colorful history and the extract from its leaves is used to improve memory and other cognitive abilities.*

REPRINTED FROM *THE HEALING HERBS* ©1991 BY MICHAEL CASTLEMAN. PERMISSION GRANTED BY RODALE PRESS, INC. EMMAUS, PA 18098.

extracts of dried herbs. Most commonly, alcohol is used to extract and preserve the active ingredients. A tincture is taken by diluting several drops in a small amount of water and drinking it. Freeze-dried herbal extracts are the most concentrated and stable of herbal preparations.

GINKGO BILOBA

The star of herbal brain boosters is the extract of the leaves of the *Ginkgo biloba* tree, which is revered for its ability to improve memory, thinking, reasoning, and general mental alertness. Ginkgo increases blood circulation through the brain to boost the brain's energy and metabolism. It is an antioxidant and facilitates the transmission of nerve signals.

Ginkgo biloba has a long, colorful history. It is the oldest tree on Earth, with fossils showing it to be more than 200 million years old. In fact, it's the last survivor of an ancient family of trees. You can say that it is the "Ishi" of the trees. (Ishi was the last surviving member of his tribe.) About 2,000 years ago, the *Ginkgo biloba* was nearly extinct; Chinese monks saved it, because they considered it to be a sacred tree. After that, they grew ginkgo in their temples. The extract from the leaves was used as a brain tonic by Chinese herbalists. The name means "bi-lobal." If you look at a ginkgo leaf, you'll see that its veins spread out in two directions, so that it looks as if the leaf is cut into two separate halves, like the lobes of the brain.

The ginkgo tree can now be found all over the world. It has won acceptance by physicians in Europe, where doctors write more than a million prescriptions a month to improve brain circulation.

Research into ginkgo's effects on humans shows that it speeds up the flow of blood and oxygen through the body and brain. It increases the manufacture of adenosine triphosphate (ATP), which is sometimes described as the "universal energy molecule." The theory is that ginkgo extract facilitates brain functioning by helping it to better metabolize glucose, which produces oxygen, the brain's main source of fuel and energy. Additionally, ginkgo keeps the brain arteries from clogging up with blood platelets, by keeping the arteries flexible so that the platelets don't collect together on the artery walls. It helps the nerve cells transmit signals from one to another. Ginkgo is a vasodilator, which means it dilates the blood vessels, especially tiny capillaries. This increased circulation helps protect the nerves from the damage that can result from a reduced supply of blood and oxygen, as often occurs with age. If all these benefits aren't enough, this astounding herb is hailed for its role as an antioxidant and its ability to improve circulation, which protects nerves from damage from reduced blood and oxygen supplies, and contributes to protection from the damage by free radicals.

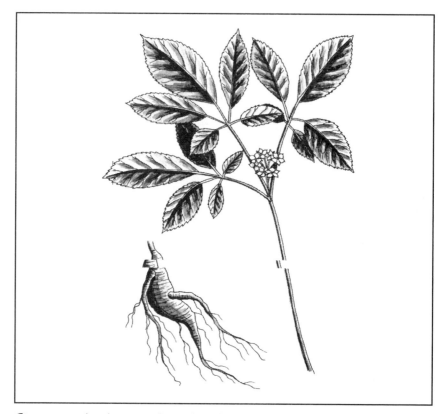

Ginseng root has been used as a health tonic in China for four thousand years.

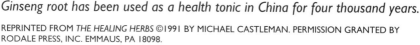

REPRINTED FROM *THE HEALING HERBS* ©1991 BY MICHAEL CASTLEMAN. PERMISSION GRANTED BY RODALE PRESS, INC. EMMAUS, PA 18098.

The active components of ginkgo leaves are flavonoid molecules called ginkgo heterosides, several terpene molecules, and organic acids, including vitamin C. The *Ginkgo biloba* extract (GBE) prepared from the leaves is marketed in Europe as Tanakan, Rokan, and Tebonin. Culture, harvesting, and extraction processes are standardized and controlled, which makes treatment more reliable and research on its effects easier.

In *The Healing Power of Herbs*, Michael Murray reviews a substantial and impressive body of research that supports traditional folk wisdom about ginkgo's beneficial impact on short-term memory, mental alertness, and general brain functioning. He says that GBE promotes an increased rate of nerve transmission, improved synthesis and turnover of cerebral neurotransmitters, and promotion of acetylcholine receptors in the hippocampus.

GBE can help people just beginning to experience a decline in their cognitive functioning due to Alzheimer's disease or other symptoms of aging. Research has shown that in aged animals GBE can normalize acetylcholine receptors in the hippocampus and increase cholinergic transmission, which helps Alzheimer's victims. But Murray cautions that GBE can delay but not prevent onset of Alzheimer's. On the other hand, he says, GBE is usually effective in reversing decline when the mental deficit is due to vascular insufficiency or depression.

Ginkgo extract is usually administered in a concentrated powdered form or in a tincture. Murray reports that at least eight days are necessary before the first effects are manifested, and that most people notice benefits within two to three weeks. Pelton says that very high doses have improved short-term memory in as little as one hour. But, generally, it is a relatively slow-acting substance. Ginkgo products are available in most health-food stores. The typical regime involves taking it three times a day, since ginkgo has a half life of about three hours, with most of the substance having dissipated after about six hours.

No side effects from the leaf extract have been reported in the scientific literature. The ginkgo fruit, on the other hand, probably should be avoided, because it causes severe allergic reactions similar to that of poison ivy and poison oak in most people who even touch it.

GINSENG

Ginseng is another superherb, sometimes called an "elixir of life," and has been used in China for more than 4,000 years as a health tonic. Even today, ginseng is considered a miracle cure-all, and is still the most widely used medicinal plant in the Orient. Although some of its uses, such as treating mental fatigue and stress, are related to mental functioning, ginseng is used to help a cornucopia of other problems, including insomnia, arthritis, TB, indigestion, high blood pressure, and cancer.

The root looks like a human, and in ancient times people imagined that God's spirit existed in it because of its human form. Consequently it is often referred to as the "root of eternal life" or the "root-of-life plant." The name itself comes from the Chinese kanji letters for *jen* and *seng*, which mean "man" and "essence," respectively. Ginseng got its botanical name, *Panax ginseng*, in 200 A.D., when a Chinese emperor called it a panacea.

Ginseng is a very shy plant and possesses many peculiar traits. It is found in unfrequented localities, and folklore has it that in the wild it must be hunted at night, when it glows under a full moon. However, wild ginseng is very rare today, even in China, and there is little evidence to support this myth. Not only does it take the root four to six years to reach maturity, but it draws so much nutrients from the soil in which it grows that another crop cannot be grown in that soil for at least ten years. Some people insist that it takes forty years for the soil to replenish.

Ginseng and its extracts come in many types and grades, depending on the source, age, parts of the root used, and preparation method used. Most valued are the old, wild, and well-formed roots. Ginseng is so popular among the Chinese that any metropolitan Chinatown of any size will have at least one store devoted solely to selling ginseng in its many forms. Highly prized old roots from the Orient can sell for more than $2,000!

The most active constituents are ginsenosides, which comprise thirteen different triterpenoidsaponins. The type and concentration of ginsenosides differs from Siberian to Korean to American ginseng.

Ginseng has its beneficial power, according to researchers, because it functions as an *adaptogen*, a term created by Dr. Brekhman, a Russian pharmacologist. Essentially, an adaptogen is a nontoxic substance that increases the body's resistance to stress and normalizes the way the body functions to bring it back into balance, which in turn helps to protect against feeling stress or fatigue.

Ginseng's effects are nonspecific. It works in a holistic way to increase resistance to adverse influences by a wide range of physical, chemical, and biochemical factors. This accounts for its broad use for many things. As a result, no matter what the problem, as an adaptogen, ginseng helps the body and the mind achieve homeostasis and balance to return to a normal condition of health. In *Longevity,* Keeton reports Doel Soejarto, a professor at University of Illinois and an expert in the study of the botanical sources of drugs, as saying that ginseng acts as both a tranquilizer and an energy booster that produces a stress-neutralizing action that is calming.

In the last few decades, extensive research has accumulated supporting the potency of ginseng and thus validating its historical reputation. Researchers have found that ginseng improves the way the mind works in several ways. It improves the brain's ability to concentrate, remember, and learn. It fights against free radicals that damage cells in the brain and elsewhere in the body, and increases circulation to the brain and to the rest of the body. Additionally, ginseng contributes indirectly to better mental functioning by normalizing the heart beat, the blood sugar, and blood pressure, by increasing endocrine activity and the metabolism rate, and by increasing the resistance to drugs, alcohol, chemotherapy, and other toxins. Ginseng improves athletic performance, reduces the amount of time needed to recover after exercising, speeds recovery from stress, helps overcome insomnia, stimulates the immune system, reduces cholesterol, and improves sexual performance. Wow!

One effect of ginseng that has withstood numerous tests of double-blind research is its antifatigue activity. For example, in a well-known Russian study, mice receiving ginseng were compared to mice without ginseng in their endurance in swimming in cold water and running up an apparently endless rope. Mice given ginseng were able to endure the "exercise" up to 183 percent longer than control mice. Other research has demonstrated that the antifatigue action results from stimulation of the central nervous system as well as from improved energy metabolism during prolonged exercise. Ginseng's amazing effects have been replicated in double-blind studies using soldiers, athletes, and nurses. For example, nurses who switched from day to night duty were tested for mental and physical performance, and rated themselves for compe-

tence, mood, and general well-being. Nurses using ginseng demonstrated higher scores on all measures as compared to those taking a
placebo.

Ginseng helps the body ward off stress. Anything that causes a
disturbance is a stressor. This includes loud noise, toxins in the
environment and produced by microorganisms, heat and cold, strong
emotional reactions, and physical injury. Ginseng increases the body's
ability to cope with stressors by acting on the adrenal glands, according
to Murray. The adrenal glands go to work during the fight-flight
response, and ginseng delays this response. Pelton points to ginseng's
ability to increase norepinephrine levels during stress. Norepinephrine
is a chemical in the brain that influences mood and memory. Low levels
result in mental fatigue and concentration problems.

Ginseng can perk up the ability to concentrate, think better, and be
more alert, because it normalizes the blood-sugar level. A drop in blood
sugar creates a condition known as *hypoglycemia,* with symptoms of
mental fatigue, confused thinking, and difficulty in concentrating. With
ginseng intake, the process is reversed, leading to greater clarity. On the
other hand, should the level of glucose in the blood be too high, ginseng
will lower the excess level because of its normalizing powers as an
adaptogen. In effect, with ginseng, you can have your cake and eat it too.
Either way, your blood sugar and other bodily functions will stay normal.
Then, too, ginseng stimulates the adrenal cortex, which results in more
ability to remember, improved learning, and even faster brain activity
to increase short-term and long-term memory.

Ginseng's effect on improving circulation to the brain contributes to
mental functioning, because when circulation declines, so does the
level of oxygen fueling the brain. According to researchers, this
improved level of blood circulation contributes to improving the functions of the hypothalamus and the pituitary glands. This improves
mental functioning, since the chemicals produced in these glands
control many of the functions in the brain.

Ginseng is available in a variety of forms in most health-food stores
and Chinese grocery stores; these include tinctures, extracts, pills,
capsules, tablets, powders, pastes, dried roots, sliced dried roots, and

granular teas. Sometimes it is mixed into wines, liquors, and chewing gums. Extracts and teas are most easily absorbed by the body. Ginseng has a bitter taste that becomes enjoyable once one gets accustomed to it. Of course, sugar and honey can sweeten it. Some people prefer to chew the root, but the root shouldn't be swallowed, since the digestive system can't break down the cellulose in it. According to Andrew Weil, ginseng must be taken regularly over a period of weeks or months to have maximum effect.

One problem with ginseng is that there is no standardization in the processing or in the potency of the products. The less-expensive roots can have very little active ingredients. Much of what is available in the American marketplace has been derived from the lower-grade roots. The serious consumer might consider consulting a professional Chinese herbalist, which would be an adventure in itself. Alternatively, many health-food-store proprietors are knowledgeable, and can help consumers judge the quality and potency of the many products available.

GOTU-KOLA AND FO-TI-TIENG

Gotu-kola is a plant found in India, China, Indonesia, Australia, the South Pacific, and areas of Africa. Although most revered for its beneficial effects on cellulite, varicose veins, wound healing, and various skin conditions, it is also known to improve mental functioning, according to Murray. He cites one study in which thirty developmentally disabled children took gotu-kola for twelve weeks. The children became more attentive and their concentration improved. Triterpenes, which are the active ingredient in gotu-kola, are mildly tranquilizing, and reduce stress and anxiety responses.

Gotu-kola is widely used in India to improve memory and longevity. Pelton says that it is a "naturally excellent neural tonic" that builds mental stamina slowly and improves nerve health. John Mann in *Secrets of Life Extension* says that herbalists and longevists swear by gotu-kola as a brain stimulant, detoxifying agent, and cell energizer.

Fo-ti-tieng, which translates from Chinese as "elixir of long life," according to Gottlieb in *Sex Drugs and Aphrodisiacs,* is a plant so similar to gotu-kola that botanists suspect it to be a geographic variant. Fo-ti-tieng was popularized by Li Chung Yun, who was born in 1677 and lived until 1933 or 256 years, according to Chinese government records. At the time of his death he was living with his twenty-fourth wife. Although these dates are just a *little* incredible, it has been established that he did live an unusually long life, and was physically vigorous until the end. He raised his own food, followed a stringent vegetarian diet, and fasted frequently. Li Chung Yun used fo-ti-tieng and ginseng regularly. The French biochemist Jules Lepine did a chemical analysis of fo-ti-tieng that revealed an alkaloid that, he claimed, had a rejuvenating effect on nerves and brain.

Gotu-kola and fo-ti-tieng can be obtained in most health-food stores powdered in capsules and tinctures. Mann prefers tea made from fresh leaves. He says that chewing a couple of leaves a day will act as a psychic energizer.

CAFFEINE

Caffeine, which acts on the dopamine system, is one of the strongest legal stimulants available. A persuasive argument can be made that it is a drug and not an herb. When taken in a refined form in over-the-counter preparations such as No-Doz, it definitely qualifies as a drug. Michael Castleman, in *The Healing Herbs*, quoted a report that noted, "If caffeine were a newly synthesized drug, its manufacturer would almost certainly have great difficulty getting it licensed under current FDA regulations. If it were licensed, it would almost certainly be available only by prescription."

In its herbal form, caffeine is found in coffee, which is consumed by millions of people daily. It is also found in tea, cola and other sodas, and in the South American drinks yerba maté and guarana. Most commonly, caffeine is taken in the form of a drink like coffee, tea, or cola.

Caffeine is highly addictive. It activates the sympathetic nervous system and makes people jumpy, anxious, and sometimes fearful. It is probably the stimulating effect that makes people believe that caffeine helps them to think and perform better. Weil believes that most people who drink coffee daily are addicted. Without morning coffee the person experiences mental and physical slowness, has problems concentrating, and is often irritable. After drinking coffee the person feels more quick-witted and able to concentrate. This common experience leads many people to conclude that caffeine is a smart drug. Actually, the opposite is true. Research reviewed by Dean and Morgenthaler showed that in controlled studies subjects performed more poorly on recall tasks.

Caffeine can also aggravate health problems. Weil recommends that caffeine be avoided by people with migraines, tremors, anxiety, insomnia, cardiovascular problems, elevated serum cholesterol, gastrointestinal disorders, urinary disorders, prostate problems, fibrocystic breast disease (there is evidence that caffeine contributes to breast cysts, for example), premenstrual syndrome, tension headaches, or seizures. Castleman cautions that chronic high-dose use can lead to *caffeinism*, a condition having the same symptoms as anxiety neurosis. These include nervousness and irritability, muscle tension, insomnia, heart palpitations, diarrhea, heartburn, and irritable stomach. (One wonders how many people in psychotherapy would be cured by simply dropping coffee from their diets.) The phenomena can be explained by looking at coffee's impact upon the noradrenaline system. Production of adrenaline and noradrenaline are stimulated by stress and unrelenting stress uses up the available noradrenaline. Coffee keeps us alert and active by activating the noradrenaline system. But, like a car running out of gas, coffee does nothing to replenish the noradrenaline it uses up. By the end of a stressful four-or-five cup of coffee day, the jitteriness and irritability experienced are signs that you're literally running on empty.

The typical dose is one or two cups in the morning or afternoon. Research indicates that drip and instant coffee do not raise cholesterol as much as coffee that has been boiled. Five cups a day has been demonstrated to double the risk of heart attack. Tea is probably a safer source. However, tea contains tannis, which irritates the digestive tract and is associated with certain cancers. This risk can be reduced by drinking tea the English way: adding milk. Milk neutralizes the tannis.

COCA

Coca is native to Peru and Bolivia, and has been successfully grown in Colombia, Jamaica, Ecuador, Brazil, Chile, Java, Ceylon, India, France, and the United States. The active substance in coca is cocaine. Although cocaine is considered a fairly dangerous hard drug, in its natural form in the coca leaf it is a gentle stimulant that has been used for centuries by the natives of South America.

LETTER FROM PRESIDENT WILLIAM MCKINLEY
Executive Mansion, Washington, June 14, 1889

My Dear Sir,
Please accept thanks on the President's behalf and on my own for your courtesy in sending a case of the celebrated Vin Mariani, with whose tonic virtues I am already acquainted, and will be happy to avail myself of in the future as occasion may require.

Very truly yours,
John Addison Porter, Secretary to the President

David Lee
Cocaine Handbook: An Essential Reference

Most early commercial products were made from the whole coca leaf. When the leaf is chewed, coca can clear the mind, elevate mood, and energize. Coca is esteemed in certain Indian groups as an aphrodisiac, and reputed to ensure longevity. In 1884, Angelo Mariani produced a wine made from coca that was wildly popular. He sent cases to physicians and fashionable connoisseurs. The recipe was secret. Mariani received and published twelve volumes of testimonials to its tonic virtues from people like Jules Verne, Sarah Bernhardt, the Czar and Czarina of Russia, Thomas Edison, and Queen Victoria. For example,

Pope Leo XIII sent a gold medal to Mariani in gratitude for the elixir made from the Divine Plant of the Incas along with a letter that said, "Rome, January 2, 1898. His Holiness has deigned to commission me to thank the distinguished donor in His holy name, and to demonstrate His gratitude in a material way as well. His Holiness does me the honour of presenting Mr. Mariani with a gold medal containing His venerable coat-of-arms" (this is, of course, a translation).

COCA: A GIFT FROM HEAVEN

Coca appears to maintain the teeth and gums in a good state of health; it keeps teeth white. The leaf is rich in vitamins, particularly thiamine, riboflavin, and C. An average daily dose of coca leaves (two ounces) supplies an Indian of the High Sierra with much of his daily vitamin requirement. Coca appears to have a beneficial influence on respiration, and is said to effect rapid cures of altitude sickness. It also rids the blood of toxic metabolites, especially uric acid. Indians say that regular use of coca promotes longevity as well. According to Indian tradition, coca was a gift from Heaven to better the lives of people on Earth.

Andrew Weil
The Green and The White
The Coca Leaf and Cocaine Papers

During this same time period, Johnstyth Pemberton, a Georgia pharmacist, developed a nonalcoholic tonic soda as a temperance drink that he called Coca-Cola. Both Vin Mariani and Coca-Cola were sold as elixirs. An 1887 advertisement for Coca-Cola called it an "intellectual beverage" and said it was "not only a delicious, exhilarating, refreshing, and invigorating beverage, but a valuable brain tonic and a cure for all nervous affections." Whether or not coca actually improves mental functioning has not been clearly established. The stimulating effect definitely makes people feel energized and provides at least an illusion of being smarter and quicker-witted.

The Indians chewed the coca leaves along with a pinch of lime from calcinated seashells. First the leaves are chewed to moisten and break them, and the stalks and strings removed. Then the lime is added a pinch at a time until the proper mixture is achieved. Eventually the chewed leaves become a "wad," is kept between the teeth and cheek, and is sucked upon. The lime interacts with the coca in such a way that the concentrated cocaine alkaloid is released. Lime is caustic, and too much will burn the mouth. The cocaine alkaloid content was not the prime factor in choice of leaves. The Indians consistently chose leaves with a lower cocaine content, but a high concentration of sweet, aromatic compounds, which gave the wad of coca better flavor.

Coca tea is another way to use coca, and probably more palatable to most people than chewing a wad. The teas do come in boxes of a dozen to twenty tea bags. The tea is made in the same manner as any tea. It provides a mild, enjoyable uplift.

We all know that cocaine, which is synthesized from coca, is an extremely strong stimulant that has high potential for abuse and that can cause serious health problems, especially cardiovascular problems. In leaf form it is difficult to overdose on coca, whether chewed or taken as a tea. Further, in this natural form, there are other natural substances that buffer the cocaine alkaloid.

CHOCOLATE: FOOD OF THE GODS

Chocolate is probably the favorite brain booster. The average American consumes 9 pounds of chocolate a year, creating a market of over $6 billion. Even though millions of people consume this addictive psychoactive, little is actually known about its pharmacology and actual effects on cognition.

Chocolate is the product of the seeds from the tropical cacao tree. Its Latin name, *Theobroma cacao L,* is a combination of the Greek words for god (*theos*) and food (*broma*)—"food of the gods." Cacao was considered the gift of Quetzoquatl, the plumed serpent god of wisdom. It was revered by the Aztecs and Mayans who consumed it in religious ceremonies. The Meso-Americans used cacao to stimulate alertness and as an aphrodisiac. Cacao beans were used as currency in trade and to pay taxes. Imagine the surprise of the Spanish conquistador Cortez, when he discovered that Aztecs valued cacao more highly than gold.

Jonathan Ott, in his fascinating polemic, *The Cacahuatl Eater*, chronicles the history, nutritional value, and psychoactive properties of chocolate. Chocolate contains proteins, vitamins, and minerals including calcium, phosphorus, iron, sodium, potassium, vitamin A, thiamine, riboflavin, and niacin. In addition, it contains theobromine and caffeine, which are alkaloids. Since theobromine is present in much larger amounts than caffeine, Ott argues that theobromine rather than caffeine is the source of the psychoactive and addictive properties of chocolate. However, Andrew Weil, in *From Chocolate to Morphine*, attributes at least some of the psychoactive properties of chocolate to the caffeine it contains.

Like caffeine, theobromine is a stimulant, yet without the "jitters" often associated with drinking coffee. Many habitual coffee users avoid coffee in the evening because it may keep them from sleeping well. Chocolate does not seem to have this kind of effect. In fact, hot cocoa is widely used as a night-time drink. Generally, children and seniors are generally discouraged from using coffee, whereas chocolate is considered so benign that it is okay.

Theobromine probably acts on the brain in a way similar to caffeine, which stimulates the central nervous system and acts on the dopamine chemistry. While caffeine is readily available in pills, theobromine is not generally used in a refined form. Instead, most people consume chocolate with sugar, cream, and other foods. Therefore the brain-stimulating effect of chocolate is that of the combination of the ingredients and their synergy with theobromine.

Like most stimulants, chocolate makes a person feel more alert and quick-witted. However, there has been little pharmacological research on theobromine and its specific measurable effects. One study in Great Britain measured improved performance of race horses dosed with theobromine. The study was done because some horses had positive results for theobromine on drug tests after having eaten cocoa bean husks. Based on these results, feeding race horses cocoa bean husks, chocolate, or theobromine in any form is illegal because it is now considered to give the horse an unfair advantage. It has not yet been scientifically proven that chocolate actually makes people smarter in terms of test scores and other performance criteria.

Theobromine, like some other brain boosters, is often described as an aphrodisiac. Chocolate is associated with romance. Chocolate candy, often in the shape of a heart, is given as a gift of love on Valentines Day and at other times as a symbol of affection. Research into the pharmacology of theobromine seems to have supported this "folk wisdom" about chocolate. In a study cited by Ott, theobromine was shown to exert a significant sexually stimulating effect on hornets.

Researchers Liebowitz and Klein proposed that the pleasant feelings we call "being in love" are stimulated by the production of a biochemical called B-phenethylamine in the brain when in the presence of the beloved. They described the jilted lover symptoms as "withdrawal" from B-phenethylamine, a condition they called "hysteroid dysphoria." Liebowitz and Klein maintain that chocolate contains significant amounts of B-phenethylamine and that this is the reason it has become associated with romance. They observe that the lovelorn often eat large amounts of chocolate and speculate that this is an attempt to substitute the B-phenethylamine in the chocolate for that produced in the brain when with one's beloved.

Andrew Weil describes people with chocolate addiction, called "chocoholics," as having symptoms different from those found in other forms of stimulant dependence. Many chocoholics are women who consume it in cyclic binges as an instant but temporary antidepressant. Besides its potential for addiction, another drawback of chocolate is that users tend to gain unwanted weight due to the large amounts of cream and sugar in most chocolate candies and desserts. Unfortunately for the chocoholics in search of love, they may eat so much chocolate that they gain unattractive weight, thereby reducing their chances at love.

Used in moderation chocolate is a pleasant brain booster. Eating chocolate is an aesthetic experience. Gourmet chocolate dishes and candies are served at parties and family events to promote warm feelings and conversation. Chocolate is used by automobile drivers and airplane pilots to stay alert. Lovers use it to heighten their attention to one another. Students eat chocolate to score better on tests and adults often eat a chocolate bar along with a cup of coffee to perform better at work. Parents often intuitively use chocolate to help their kids learn. Not only does the theobromine in the chocolate stimulate the brain to increase learning, but the wonderful sweet chocolate taste, as well as its feel in the mouth, rewards the kids for learning.

GREEN FOODS

In recent years there has been increasing interest in "green foods," which include wheat grass and a variety of microalgae.

WHEAT AND BARLEY GRASS

Juiced wheat and barley grasses have become nutritional drinks among health food enthusiasts. We've all seen cows and horses chomping on grass, which is their primary food. It's amazing to think that thick, juicy steaks come from Black Angus fed nothing but grass. But as it turns out, grass is very nutritious. Wheat grass is a rich source of vitamins A, B, C, and E, which are all antioxidants. Recall that antioxidants slow brain aging by destroying free radicals. Grasses contain all of the known minerals and are especially rich in calcium, phosphorous, iron, potassium, sulfur, cobalt, and zinc. Many of these minerals are essential for the brain to function well.

As we all know, grass has a high chlorophyll content, which gives it its green color. Many experts call chlorophyll "nature's healer" because it produces an unfavorable environment for bacterial growth in the body and helps eliminate toxins. Dr. Bernard Jensen, author of *Health Magic Through Chlorophyll*, states that chlorophyll can be used as an antidote to pesticides and can help eliminate drug deposits from the body. Other research performed by the U. S. Army showed that chlorophyll-rich foods may be effective in decreasing the effects of radiation. Toxins of these sort generate free radicals that attack brain cells. All indications are that chlorophyll acts as a toxin cleanser.

Humans don't have the ability to digest grass. To get the nutritional benefits, the grass must be juiced. A typical serving is usually about one to four ounces. Some people experience nausea when they begin using it. Grass enthusiasts claim that this is due to its powerful cleansing properties and the release of toxins in the system. They recommend that people start with one ounce servings and gradually increase their intake to four ounces.

Once juiced, grass is not stable and will go bad quickly. It should be used within about ten minutes of juicing. Cut grass can be stored in plastic containers in a refrigerator without spoiling for about a week. When frozen, grass will keep for longer periods but does lose some of its nutrition.

MICROALGAE

Microalgae are single-celled plants that grow in fresh water. We've all seen them. They are that strange green "slime" growing on ponds in the woods. Spirulina and chlorella are the most widely used food algae. Seaweeds are another form of algae and have been used in food dishes in the Orient for thousands of years. In the early 1950s researchers began to investigate the use of microalgae as a source of food and medicine for humans. In the years since, chlorella production has grown into a $100 million a year industry in Japan. Spirulina is most commonly used in the United States.

Like grass, algae is high in chlorophyll. As you might guess from its name, chlorella is the richest source of chlorophyll available for human nutrition. Whereas alfalfa contains about 2% chlorophyll, chlorella is about 76% chlorophyll. One of the most remarkable nutritional qualities of microalgae is its high protein content. It contains more protein than beef or other meats; more protein than soybeans, which are very high in protein. Algae is very rich in amino acids. As you can see in the table, Sun Chlorella, produced in Japan, contains glutamic acid, which is essential for neutralizing ammonia metabolic waste in the brain. It also contains arginine, which is converted into spermine in the body. Low levels of spermine are associated with senility and memory loss.

INGREDIENTS IN SUN-CHLORELLA "A" PER 100 GRAMS

Amino Acids

Lysine	3.46 w/w%
Histidine	1.29 w/w%
Arginine	3.64 w/w%
Aspartic acid	5.20 w/w%
Threonine	2.70 w/w%
Serine	2.78 w/w%
Glutamic acid	6.29 w/w%
Proline	2.93 w/w%
Glycine	3.40 w/w%
Alanine	4.80 w/w%
Cystine	0.38 w/w%
Valine	3.64 w/w%
Methionine	1.45 w/w%
Isoleucine	2.63 w/w%
Leucine	5.26 w/w%
Tryosine	2.09 w/w%
Phenylalanine	3.08 w/w%
Ornithine	0.06 w/w%
Tryptophan	0.59 w/w%

Fatty Acids

Unsaturated	81.8%
Saturated	18.2%

Vitamins and Minerals

Vitamin A	55,500IU/100g
B-carotene	180.8 mg
Chlorophyll a	1,469 mg
Chlorophyll b	613 mg
Thiamine	1.5 mg
Riboflavin	4.8 mg
Vitamin B_6	1.7 mg
Vitamin B_{12}	125.9 mcg
Vitamin C	15.6 mg
Vitamin E	>1 IU
Niacin (B_3)	23.8 mg
Pantothenic acid (B_5)	1.3 mg
Folic acid	26.9 mcg
Biotin	191.6 mcg
Para-amino-benzoic acid	0.6 mcg
Inositol	165 mg
Calcium	205 mg
Iodine	0.6 mg
Magnesium	315 mg
Iron	167 mg
Zinc	71 mg
Copper	0.08 mg

SUN-CHLORELLA "A" is a product of Sun Chlorella Company.

*w/w = wet weight

Dhyana Bewicke
Chlorella: The Emerald Food

Phenylalanine, which is a popular ingredient in smart drinks, is found in microalgae as well. Phenylalanine is important in the production of the neurotransmitters norepinephrine and dopamine.

A look at the list of vitamins and minerals in chlorella reveals many that are important for optimal brain functioning. Specifically, vitamins A, B, C, and E are antioxidants that destroy the free radicals. Finally, chlorella is high in unsaturated fats and low in saturated fats which is what Andrew Weil recommends. Recall that brain cells are 60 percent fat.

Algae grows in fresh water ponds. The purity of the water is important because, as it grows, the algae absorbs nutrients from the water. If there are toxins in the water, they will be absorbed as well. In the late 1970s wild spirulina was harvested from contaminated ponds and sold commercially. A number of people suffered gastrointestinal distress and spirulina developed a bad name as a result. Sun Chlorella is cultivated in stainless steel vats and harvested in sterile conditions in Japan. Super Blue Green™ is a trade marked name for *Aphanizomenon flos-aquae*, which they claim is not spirulina but another strain of algae cultivated on the Upper Klamath Lake in Oregon. The nutritional analysis for Super Blue Green is very similar to that for Sun Chlorella except that it also contains 34 mg. of choline. Choline is converted in the body into the neurotransmitter acetylcholine, which is important for memory formation and recall. One of their products, which they call Omega Sun™, is touted as "energy for the mind" and a boost for demanding mental pursuits in which increased memory and mental clarity are desired. The cell wall of the algae is broken and removed in the preparation of this product, leaving the "heart" of the algae, which is high in amino acids. They claim that in this form the amino acids can cross the brain-blood barrier to enter the brain cells directly. Chlorella, which has an undigestible cell wall, has its wall removed in all chlorella products. The nucleus of the chlorella contains a substance called "chlorella growth factor," which is extracted and sold as a thick green liquid super-powered health food. Its amino acid content is even higher than the standard chlorella products. It was discovered by Dr. Fujimaki of the People's Scientific Research Center at Koganei in Tokyo who claims that it stimulates the immune system and accelerates the growth and development of new cells, including brain cells.

OTHER BRAIN-BOOSTING HERBS

In *The Handbook of Alternatives to Chemical Medicine,* Jackson and Teague cite several herbs as useful brain tonics. They say that common sage supplies oxygen to the brain, and recommend sage tea to revitalize the brain and improve concentration. Mental fatigue and forgetfulness can be relieved by a tea made from mugwort and rosemary. Another tea, yerba maté, is a stimulant that acts like caffeine and can stimulate the intellect. Chamomile is a popular tea that Jackson and Teague say stimulates the brain and dispells weariness.

It is probably true that less scientific research has been performed in the West on the effects of herbs than on the effects of drugs, vitamins, minerals, and other nutrients. As we noted earlier, in our culture, herbs have been used almost exclusively to spice foods, and the active substances in herbs have generally not been isolated. However, the testimonies of those who use herbs as brain boosters, the long traditions of folk and medicinal uses of herbs in other cultures, and their relative harmlessness make herbs a promising area both for personal experimentation and for future scientific research.

BIBLIOGRAPHY

NEWSLETTERS

Brain/Mind Bulletin, 4047 San Rafael, Los Angeles, CA 90065;
213-342-9937.

*Forefront Health Investigations: The Journal of Theoretical and Applied Health
Technologies,* Steven Wm. Fowkes, Editor, MegaHealth Society,
Box 60637, Palo Alto, CA 94306; 415-949-0919.

Intelli-Scope: The Newsletter of the Designer Foods Network, Smart Products,
870 Market Street, Suite 1262, San Francisco, CA 94102; 415-981-3334.

Life Extension Report, Saul Kent, Publisher, Box 229120, Hollywood,
FL 33022; 305-966-4886.

Nootropic News, John Leslie, Editor, P.O. Box 177, Camarillo, CA 93011.

*Smart Drug News: The Newsletter of the Cognitive Enhancement Research
Institute,* CERI, Box 4029-4002, Menlo Park, CA 94026; 415-321-2374;
Fax 415-323-3864.

BOOKS AND ARTICLES

Andrews, G. and D. Solomon, *The Coca Leaf and Cocaine Papers,* Harcourt
Brace Jovanovich, New York, NY, 1975.

Bewicke, Dhyana, and Beverly Potter, *Chlorella: The Emerald Food,* Ronin
Publishing, Berkeley, CA, 1984.

Bishop, Katherine, "Baby Boomers Fight Aging by Dropping Acid (Amino),"
The New York Times, June 10, 1992, page B-1.

Brown, David Jay, "On Curing...and the FDA's War on Smart Drugs," *High
Times,* September, 1992, page 38.

Calbom, Cherie and Maureen Keane, *Juicing for Life,* Avery Publishing Group,
Garden City Park, NY, 1992.

Castleman, Michael, *The Healing Herbs*, Rodale Press, Emmaus, PA, 1991.

Dean, Ward, and John Morgenthaler, *Smart Drugs & Nutrients*, B & J Publications, Santa Cruz, CA, 1991.

Dean, Ward, *Biological Aging Measurement: Clinical Applications*, The Center for Bio-Gerontology, Pensacola, FL, 1992.

Dilman, Vladimir M. and Ward Dean. *The Neuroendocrine Theory of Aging and Degenerative Disease*, Center for Bio-Gerontology, Pensacola, FL, 1992.

Dimond, Marian. *Enriching Heredity: The Impact of the Environment on the Anatomy of the Brain*, The Center for Bio-Gerontology, Pensacola, FL, 1992.

The Directory of Life Extension Nutrients and Drugs, Life Extension International, Hollywood, FL, 1992.

The Directory of Life Extension Doctors, Life Extension Foundation, Ft. Lauderdale, FL.

Directory of Mail Order Suppliers, *Nootropic News*, Camarillo, CA.

Erdmann, Robert, *The Amino Revolution*, Simon & Schuster, New York, 1987.

Farley, Christopher John, "Smart Drugs Challenge Conventional Wisdom," *USA Today*, Life Section, September 26, 1991.

Gottlieb, Adam, *Sex Drugs and Aphrodisiacs*, Ronin Publishing, Berkeley, CA, 1993.

Hauer, Christina, "An Overdose of Pessimism: What a Top Analyst Thinks Has Hit the Drug Group," *Barron's*, May 4, 1992.

Hoffer, Abram and Morton Walker, *Smart Nutrients: A Guide to Nutrients that Can Enhance Intelligence and Reverse Senility*, Avery Publishing, Garden City Park, NY, 1993.

Jackson, Mildred and Terri Teague, *The Handbook of Alternatives to Chemical Medicine*, Lawton Teague, Oakland, CA, 1975.

Joy, Dan, "Introduction to the Psychedelic Encyclopedia," in Stafford, Peter *Psychedelic Encyclopedia*, Ronin Publishing, Berkeley, CA, 1992.

Keeton, Kathy, *Longevity: The Science of Staying Young*, Viking Penguin, New York, NY, 1992.

Kessler, David, *Caring for the Elderly: Reshaping Health Policy*, John Hopkins University Press.

Lee, David, *Cocaine Handbook: An Essential Reference*, And/Or Press, Berkeley, CA, 1981.

Mann, John A., *Secrets of Life Extension: How to Halt or Reverse the Aging Process and Live a Long and Healthy Life*, And/Or Press, Berkeley, CA, 1980.

Mark, Vernon, and Jeffrey Mark, *Reversing Memory Loss: Proven Methods for Regaining, Strengthening, and Preserving Memory*, Houghton Mifflin Company, Boston, MA, 1992.

Morgenthaler, John, and Steven Wm. Fowkes, *Stop the FDA: Save Your Health Freedom*, Health Freedom Publications, Milbrae, CA, 1992.

Morgenthaler, John, "New Drugs That Make You Smarter," *Mondo 2000*, January, 1991.

Mowrey, Daniel B., *The Scientific Validation of Herbal Medicine*, Cormorant Books, Lehi, UT, 1986.

Mowrey, Daniel, B., *Next Generation Herbal Medicine*, Cormorant Books, Lehi, UT, 1988.

Murray, Michael, *The 21st Century Herbal*, Vita-Line, Bellevue, WA, 1987.

Ott, Jonathan, *The Cacahuatl Eater: Ruminations of An Unabashed Chocolate Addict*, Natural Products Co, Vashon, WA, 1985.

Pearson, Durk, and Sandy Shaw, *Life Extension: A Practical Scientific Approach*, Warner Books, 1982.

Pelton, Ross, *Mind Foods and Smart Pills: A Sourcebook for the Vitamins, Herbs, and Drugs That Can Increase Intelligence, Improve Memory, and Prevent Brain Aging*, Doubleday, New York, NY, 1989.

Robbins, Cynthia. "The Ecstatic Cybernetic Amino Acid Test," *Image Magazine*, February 16, 1992, pages 11–29.

Rosenfeld, Albert. *Pro-Longevity II: An Updated Report on the Scientific Aspects of Adding Good Years To Life,* Henry Holt, New York, NY, 1985.

Schlesser, Jerry L., *Drugs Available Abroad,* Gale Research, Detroit, MI, 1991.

Scott, Gini Graham, *Success in Multi-Level Marketing,* Prentice Hall (Simon & Schuster), Englewood, NJ, 1992.

Stein, Irene, *Royal Jelly: The New Guide to Nature's Richest Health Food,* Thorsons Publishers Ltd., Wellingborough, Northamptonshire, England, 1989.

Weil, Andrew and Winifred Rosen, *From Chocolate To Morphine: Everything You Need To Know About Mind-Altering Drugs,* Revised Edition, Houghton Mifflin Co, Boston, MA, 1993.

Weil, Andrew, *Natural Health, Natural Medicine: A Comprehensive Manual for Wellness and Self-Care,* Houghton Mifflin Company, Boston, MA, 1990.

Wolf, Gary, "Smart Drugs," *S F Weekly,* March 20, 1991, page 13.

Zeman, Ned, "Through the Looking Glass: A British Dance Craze Has California Raving," *Newsweek,* April 27, 1992, page 54.

APPENDIX A

DIRECTORY OF LIFE EXTENSION DOCTORS

Compiled by The Life Extension Foundation

THE LIFE EXTENSION FOUNDATION

The Life Extension Foundation provides monthly updates on antiaging breakthroughs throughout the world. This information is five to ten years ahead of conventional medicine.

The Foundation was the first organization to introduce Americans to the Japanese drug *coenzyme Q10 (CoQ10)*. In 1983, the Foundation warned its members about the dangers of supplemental iron because of strong evidence linking iron to increased rates of cancer, heart disease, and Parkinson's disease. The information the Foundation published in the early 1980s is not accepted by mainstream medicine as being scientifically valid.

The Life Extension Foundation also provides its members with sources of advanced antiaging drugs and intelligence enhancing compounds from around the world. Years before the FDA approved deprenyl in the United States, the Foundation was assisting its members in obtaining deprenyl from low-cost sources in Europe.

Members of the Foundation also gain access to The Life Extension Buyer's Club, which provides access to the latest antiaging therapies at a small markup over the actual cost of the product.

The Life Extension Foundation is a nonprofit, tax-exempt organization. To receive a free issue of the Foundation's newsletter, call them at 1-800-841-5433 or (305) 966-4886, or write to The Life Extension Foundation, P.O. Box 229120, Hollywood, FL 33022.

ALABAMA

Birmingham
- Glenwood Mental Health Svc.,
  150 Glenwood Lane, Birmingham, AL 35243, (205) 969-2880
- P. Gus J. Prosch Jr., MD,
  759 Valley St., Birmingham, AL 35226, (205) 823-6180

Huntsville
- George Gray, MD,
  204 Lowe Bldg. 2, Ste. 7, Huntsville, AL 35801, (205) 533-4464
- Pat Hamm, MD,
  6502 Sheri Dr., NW, Huntsville, AL 35806, (205) 721-9696

Tuscaloosa
- Humphrey Osmond, MD, Bryce Nova Program,
  200 University Blvd., Tuscaloosa, AL 35401, (205) 759-0416

ALASKA

Anchorage

- Sandra Denton, MD,
  615 E. 82nd Ave., Ste. 300, Anchorage, AK 99518, (907) 344-7775
- F. Russell Manuel, MD,
  4200 Lake Otis Blvd., #304, Anchorage, AK 99508, (907) 562-7070
- Robert Rowen, MD,
  615 E. 82nd Ave., Ste. 300, Anchorage, AK 99518, (907) 344-7775

Soldotna

- Paul G. Isaak, MD,
  Box 219, Soldotna, AK 99669, (907) 262-9341

Wasilla

- Robert E. Martin, MD,
  P.O. Box 870710, Wasilla, AK 99687, (907) 376-5284

ARIZONA

Lake Havasu City

- Francis J. Woo Jr., MD,
  60 Riviera Drive, Lk. Havasu City, AZ 86403, (602) 453-3330

Parker

- S.W. Meyer, DO,
  332 River Front Dr., P.O. Box 1870, Parker, AZ 85344, (602) 669-8911

Phoenix

- Lloyd D. Armold, DO,
  4025 W. Bell Rd., Ste. 3, Phoenix, AZ 85023, (602) 939-8916
- Abram Ber, MD,
  20635 N. Cave Creek Rd., Phoenix, AZ 85024, (602) 279-3795
- Janice Bebe Dorn, MD, PHD,
  4647 N. 32nd St., #250, Phoenix, AZ 85018, (602) 224-9277
- Dharma Singh Khalsa, MD,
  Univ. of Arizona Medical School, Dept. of Pain, Stress & Longevity, Maricopa Medical Center, 2601 E. Roosevelt, Phoenix, AZ 85010, (602) 267-5141
- Stanley R. Olsztyn, MD,
  Whitton Place, 3610 N. 44th St., Ste. 210, Phoenix, AZ 85018, (602) 954-0811

ARKANSAS

Dumas

- Robert A. Hoagland, MD,
  145 W. Waterman, Dumas, AR 71639, (501) 382-4878

Leslie

- Melissa Taliaferro, MD,
  Cherry Street, P.O. Box 400, Leslie, AR 72645, (501) 447-2599

Little Rock

- Norbert J. Becquet, MD,
  115 W. Sixth St., Little Rock, AR 72201, (501) 375-4419

Pine Bluff
- Aubrey Worrell, MD,
  3900 Hickory, Pine Bluff, AR 71603, (501) 535-8200

Springdale
- Doty Murphy III, MD,
  812 Dorman, Springdale, AR 72764, (501) 756-3251

CALIFORNIA

Albany
- Ross B. Gordon, MD,
  405 Kains Ave., Albany, CA 94706, (415) 526-3232

Bakersfield
- Ralph Seibly, MD,
  1311 Columbus St., Bakersfield, CA 93305, (805) 832-3830

Baldwin Park
- Kenneth Tye, MD,
  141000 Francisquito Avenue, Suite 9, Baldwin Park, CA 91706, (818) 960-6588

Berkeley
- Stephen Langer, MD,
  3031 Telegraph Ave, #230, Berkeley, CA 94705, (510) 548-7384
- Timothy J. Smith, MD,
  2635 Regent Street, Berkeley, CA 94704, (510) 548-8022

Beverly Hills
- Bronk, DC,
  206 S. Robertson Blvd., Beverly Hills, CA 90211, (213) 659-3870

Brea
- Edgar Lucidi, MD,
  410 W. Central Ave., Brea, CA 92621, (714) 879-9500

Burbank
- Robert Gibbons, DC,
  3808 Riverside Dr., #105, Burbank, CA 91505, (818) 563-1990

Campbell
- Carol A. Shamlin, MD,
  621 E. Campbell, Ste. 11A, Campbell, CA 95008, (408) 378-7970

Chico
- Eva Jalkotzy, MD,
  156 Eaton Rd. #E, Chico, CA 95926, (916) 893-3080

Concord
- John T. Toth, MD,
  2299 Bacon St., Ste. 10, Concord, CA 94520, (510) 682-5660

Corte Madera
- Michael Rosenbaum, MD,
  45 San Clement Dr., Suite B-130, Corte Madera, CA 94925, (415) 927-9450

Costa Mesa
- Stanley Hansen, MD, FAPA,
  440 Fair Drive, Ste. K, Costa Mesa, CA 92626, (714) 557-5500

Cotati
- Anu de Monterice, MD,
  680-682 E. Cotati Ave., Cotati, CA 94931, (707) 795-2141

Covina
- James Privitera, MD,
  105 No. Grandview Ave., Covina, CA 91723, (818) 966-1618

Cupertino
- Carl Ebother, MD,
  20360 Town Center Ln., #5G, Cupertino, CA 95014

Del Mar
- Harold H. Bloomfield, MD,
  1011 Camino Del Mar, Suite 234, Del Mar, CA 92014, (619) 481-7102
- Ronald M. Lesko, DO, MPH,
  13983 Mango Drive, Suite #102, Del Mar, CA 92014, (619) 259-2444

El Cajon
- William J. Saccoman, MD,
  505 N. Mollison Ave., Suite 103, El Cajon, CA 92021, (619) 440-3838

Encino
- A. Leonard Klepp, MD,
  16311 Ventura Blvd., #725, Encino, CA 91436, (818) 981-5511

Eureka
- Muriel Bramwell,
  2435 Chester St., Eureka, CA 95501, (707) 443-2306

Fresno
- David J. Edwards, MD,
  360 S. Clovis Ave., Fresno, CA 93727, (209) 251-5066

Grand Terrace
- Bruce Halstead, MD,
  22807 Barton Road, Grand Terrace, CA 92324, (714) 783-2773

Hayward
- Robert Buckley, MD,
  1320 Apple, #203, Hayward, CA 94541, (415) 886-7002

Hollywood
- James Julian, MD,
  1654 Cahuenga Blvd., Hollywood, CA 90028, (213) 467-5555 or, (213) 466-0126

Huntington Beach
- Joan M. Resk, DO,
  18821 Delaware St., #203, Huntington Beach, CA 92648, (714) 842-5591

Irvine
- Bruce Battleson, MD,
  18124 Culver Dr. #G, Irvine, CA 92715, (714) 786-3433

Kentfield
- Carolyn Albrecht, MD,
  10 Wolfe Grade, Kentfield, CA 94904, Retired

La Jolla
- Dr. Thomas A. Munson,
  750 Bon Air Pl, La Jolla, CA 92037, (619) 454-0780

La Mesa
- John C. Dodgen, MD,
  5185 Comanche Drive #A, La Mesa, CA 92116, (619) 464-8924

Lake Forest
- David A. Steenblock, DO,
  22706 Aspen St., #501, Lake Forest, CA 92630, (714) 770-9616

Lawndale
- Southwestern Medical Group,
  15603 Hawthorne Blvd., Lawndale, CA 90260, (213) 644-1144

Laytonville
- Eugene D. Finkle, MD,
  50 Branscomb Road, Laytonville, CA 95454, (707) 984-6151

Long Beach
- H.R. Casdorph, MD, Ph.D.,
  1703 Termino Ave., Suite 201, Long Beach, CA 90804, (310) 597-8716

Los Altos
- Robert F. Cathcart III, MD,
  127 Second St., Los Altos, CA 94022, (415) 949-2822
- Susan M. Lark, MD,
  101 State St., #441, Los Altos, CA 94022, (415) 964-7268
- Claude J. Marquette, MD,
  5050 El Camino Real, #110, Los Altos, CA 94022-1526

Los Angeles
- Laszlo Belenyessy, MD,
  12732 Washington Blvd. #D, Los Angeles, CA 90066, (213) 822-4614
- Wes Burgess, PHD, MD,
  1990 S. Bundy Dr. #790, Los Angeles, CA 90025, (310) 207-8448
- Ray Fisch, Ph.D.,
  Nutritional Counselor, 443 S. Barrington Ave., Suite #10, Los Angeles, CA 90049,
  (310) 471-1365
- M. Jahangiri, MD,
  2156 South Santa Fe, Los Angeles, CA 90058, (213) 587-3218
- Jekot, MD,
  8474 W. 3 St., #204, Los Angeles, CA 90048, (213) 655-5900
- David Katzim, MD,
  Westwood Medical Group, 12278 Canna Road, Los Angeles, CA 90049, (310) 826-2127
- Joan Priestley, MD,
  7080 Hollywood Blvd., Suite 603, Los Angeles, CA 90028
- Harvey Ross, MD,
  7060 Hollywood Blvd., Los Angeles, CA 90028, (213) 446-8330
- Priscilla Slagle, MD,
  12301 Wilshire #300, Los Angeles, CA 90025, (213) 826-0175

Los Gatos
- Carl Ebnother, MD,
  118 Henning Court, Los Gatos, CA 95030, (415) 969-0708
- Dr. Bert Rettner,
  221 Almendra Ave., Los Gatos, CA 95030, (408) 354-2300

- R.O. Waiton, MD, DO,
  221 Almendra Avenue, Los Gatos, CA 95030, (408) 354-2300

Malibu

- Jesse Hanley, MD,
  23410 Civic Center Way, Malibu, CA 90265, (213) 456-1972

Mariposa

- Robert Casanas, MD,
  4979 Highway 140, Box 129, Mariposa, CA 95338, (208) 742-6606

Mission Hills

- Lusher, MD,
  14935 Rinaldi, Mission Hills, CA 91345, (213) 821-7658

Mission Viejo

- Dynastat Medical Group,
  25356 Malia Ct., Mission Viejo, CA 92691

Monrovia

- C. Fred Hering III, MD,
  212-A W. Foothill Blvd., Monrovia, CA 91016, (818) 357-2226

Monterey

- Lon B. Work, MD,
  841 Foam St., #D, Monterey, CA 93940, (408) 655-0215

Newport Beach

- Lee-Benner, MD,
  360 San Miguel Dr., #208, Newport Beach, CA 92660, (714) 720-9022
- Julian Whitaker, MD,
  4400 MacArthur Blvd., Suite 630, Newport Beach, CA 92660, (714) 851-1550

Northridge

- William T. Duffy, DO,
  8349 Reseda Blvd., #D, Northridge, CA 91324, (818) 349-4164

North Hollywood

- David Freeman, MD,
  11311 Camarillo St., #103, North Hollywood, CA 91602, (818) 985-1103
- Douglas Hunt, MD,
  10738 Riverside Dr., #C, North Hollywood, CA 91602, (818) 509-9955

Oakland

- Robert Wm. Tufft, Sr., MD,
  411-30th Street Suite #208, Oakland, CA 94609, (415) 444-2155

Orange

- Gerald S. Brodie, MD,
  228 S. Tustin Avenue, Orange, CA 92666, (714) 532-1678
- Greg Wolf, MD,
  777 S. Main, #99, Orange, CA 92668, (714) 541-3321

Oxnard

- Mohamed Moharram, MD,
  300 W. 5th St., Ste. B, Oxnard, CA 93030, (805) 483-2355

Pacific Palisades

- Hyla Cass, MD,
  1608 Michael Lane, Pacific Palisades, CA 90272, (310) 456-5432

Palm Desert
- David H. Tang, MD,
  74133 El Paso, #6, Palm Desert, CA 92260, (619) 341-2113

Palm Springs
- Sean Degnan, MD,
  2825 Tahquitz McCallum, Suite 200, Palm Springs, CA 92262, (619) 320-4292

Palo Alto
- Dr. Alan Brauer, Brauer Medical Center,
  630 University Ave., Palo Alto, CA 94301, (415) 329-8001
- William Sayer, MD,
  145 N. California Ave., Palo Alto, CA 94301

Porterville
- John B. Park, MD,
  131 East Mill Ave., Porterville, CA 93527, (209) 781-6224

Rancho Mirage
- Vincent Forshan, MD,
  39700 Bob Hope Dr, #301, Rancho Mirage, CA 92270, (619) 340-2141

Reseda
- Llona Abraham, MD,
  19231 Victoria Blvd., Reseda, CA 91335, (818) 345-8721

Rialto
- Clemens A. Hackethal, MD,
  1766 North Riverside Ave., Rialto, CA 92376, (714) 875-8845

San Diego
- Aline Fournier, DO,
  10969 Scripps Ranch Blvd., San Diego, CA 92131, (619) 774-6991
- Lawrence H. Taylor, MD,
  3330 Third Ave., Ste. 402, San Diego, CA 92103, (619) 296-2952

San Francisco
- Richard A. Kunin, MD,
  2698 Pacific Ave., San Francisco, CA 94115, (415) 346-2500
- Paul Lynn, MD,
  345 W. Portal Ave., San Francisco, CA 94127, (415) 566-1000
- Denise Mark, MD,
  345 W. Portal Ave., San Francisco, CA 94127, (415) 566-1000
- Daniel Martell, MD,
  16537 Franklin, #101, San Francisco, CA 94109, (415) 885-2552
- Gary S. Ross, MD,
  500 Sutter, #300, San Francisco, CA 94102, (415) 398-0555

San Jose
- Cantwell, MD,
  386 Monroe St., #1, San Jose, Ca 95128, (408) 248-1414

San Leandro
- Steven H. Gee, MD,
  595 Estudillo St., San Leandro, CA 94577, (415) 483-5881
- Stephen Levine, Ph.D.,
  400 Preda St., San Leandro, CA 94577, (415) 639-4572

San Marcos
- William C. Kubitschek, MD,
  1194 Calle Maria, San Marcos, CA 92069, (619) 744-6991

Santa Ana
- Robert B. Gold, DO,
  1220 Hemlock Way, Suite 103, Santa Ana, CA 92704, (714) 556-GOLD
- Ramon Scruggs, MD,
  1220 W. Hemlock Way, Suite 203, Santa Ana, CA 92707, (714) 549-8456

Santa Barbara
- H.J. Hoegerman, MD,
  101 W. Arrellaga, Ste. D, Santa Barbara, CA 93101, (805) 963-1824
- Mohamed Moharram, MD,
  101 W. Arrellaga, Ste. B, Santa Barbara, CA 93101, (805) 965-5229

Santa Maria
- Donald Reiner, MD,
  1414-D South Miller, Santa Maria, CA 93454, (805) 925-0961

Santa Monica
- Hyla Cass, MD,
  2730 Wilshire Blvd. #302, Santa Monica, CA 90403, (310) 453-4339
- Martin, DC,
  2212 Oak St., Suite 2, Santa Monica, CA 90405, (310) 452-7640
- Michael Rosenbaum, MD,
  2730 Wilshire Blvd., Suite 110, Santa Monica, CA 90403, (310) 453-4424
- Murray Susser, MD,
  2730 Wilshire Blvd., #110, Santa Monica, CA 90403, (310) 453-4424
- Karlis Ullis, MD,
  Medical Director, 1457 Stanford Street, Suite 6, Santa Monica, CA 90404,
  (310) 829-1990

Santa Rosa
- Thomas Collins,
  DC, 4737 Sonoma Hwy., Santa Rosa, CA 95409, (707) 538-3554
- Hollis L. Stavn,
  P.O. Box 637, Santa Rosa, CA 95402, (916) 527-9137
- Robert Yee, MD,
  3317 Chanate Rd. #2d, Santa Rosa, CA 95404, (707) 544-6891

Smith River
- James D. Schuler, MD,
  P.O. Box 297, Smith River, CA 95567, (707) 487-3405

Soquel
- Randy Baker, MD,
  2955 Park Avenue, Soquel, CA 95073, (408) 476-1886

Stanton
- William J. Goldwag, MD,
  7499 Cerritos Ave., Stanton, CA 90680, (714) 827-5180

Studio City
- Charles E. Law Jr., MD,
  3959 Laurel Canyon Blvd., Suite I, Studio City, CA 91604, (818) 761-1661

Tarzana
- Melvyn Werbach, MD,
  4751 Viviana Dr., Tarzana, CA 90505, (818) 996-6110

Torrance
- Anita Millen, MD,
  1010 Crenshaw Blvd., Suite 170, Torrance, CA 90501, (213) 320-1132
- Woodrow Weiss, MD,
  3661 Torrance Blvd., Torrance, CA 90503, (213) 544-6891
- David Wong, MD,
  3250 W. Lomita Blvd., Suite 209, Torrance, CA 90505, (213) 326-8625

Tustin
- William Bryce, MD,
  1254 Irvine Blvd., #160, Tustin, CA 92680, (714) 544-3900

Van Nuys
- Frank Mosler, MD,
  14428 Gilmore St., Van Nuys, CA 91401, (818) 785-7425

Walnut Creek
- Alan Shifman Charles, MD,
  1414 Maria Lane, Walnut Creek, CA 94596, (510) 937-3331

West Los Angeles
- Thomas M. Brod, MD,
  12304 Santa Monica Blvd., Suite 210, West Los Angeles, CA 90025, (213) 207-3337

Woodland Hills
- Alexander Sinavsky, MD,
  22381 Algunas Rd., Woodland Hills, CA 91364, (818) 883-9079

COLORADO

Colorado Springs
- James R. Fish, MD,
  3030 N. Hancock, Colorado Springs, CO 80907, (719) 471-2273
- George Juetersonke, DO,
  5455 N. Union Blvd., #200, Colorado Springs, CO 80918, (719) 528-1960

Denver
- Christopher J. Hussar, DO,
  Grassroots Health Spa, 2222 E. 18th Avenue, Denver, CO 80206, (303) 333-3733
- Thomas Lawrence, DC,
  Grassroots Health Spa, 2222 E. 18th Avenue, Denver, CO 80206, (303) 333-3733

Englewood
- John H. Altshuler, MD,
  Greenwood Exec. Park, Building 10, 7485 E. Peakview Ave., Englewood CO 80111,
  (303) 740-7771

Grand Junction
- William L. Reed, MD,
  591-25 Road, Ste. A-4, Grand Junction, CO 81505, (303) 241-3631

CONNECTICUT

Bristol

- Tom Laga, PHD,
  59 Adeline Ave, Bristol, CT 06010

Norwalk

- Marshall Mandell, MD,
  3 Brush Street, Norwalk, CT 06850, (203) 838-4706

Orange

- Robban Sica-Cohen, MD,
  Alan R. Cohen, M.D., 325 Post Road, Orange, CT 06477, (203) 799-7733

DISTRICT OF COLUMBIA

Washington

- Paul Beals, MD,
  2639 Connecticut Ave. N.W., Suite 100, Washington, D.C. 20037, (202) 332-0370

FLORIDA

Altamonte Springs

- Joya Lynn Schoen, M.D.,
  341 N. Maitland Ave., Suite 200, Atlamonte Springs, FL 32751, (407) 644-2729

Arcadia

- Jarrett C. Black, MD, PA,
  House of Black Bldg., Rt. 8 Hwy. 70 Box 94-A, Arcadia, FL 33821, (813) 494-6215

Boca Raton

- Leonard Haimes, MD,
  Metabolic Health Systems, 7300 N. Federal Hwy., #107, Boca Raton, FL 33487,
  (407) 994-3868
- Albert F. Robbins, DO,
  400 S. Dixie Hwy., Boca Raton, FL 33432, (407) 395-3282

Crystal River

- Carlos F. Gonzalez, MD,
  9030 W. Fort Island Trail, Suite 1, Crystal River, FL 32629, (904) 795-4711
- Eileen O'Ferrell Adams, MD,
  P.O. Box 820, Crystal River, FL 32629, (904) 795-9406

Davie

- Robert P. Ellis, PHD,
  1809 S.W. 81st Terr., Davie, FL 33324

Fort Lauderdale

- Ervin Barr, DO,
  2350 W. Oakland Park Blvd., Ft. Lauderdale, FL 33311, (305) 731-8080
- Edmond Kuell, LN,
  3012 Granda St., #5, Ft. Lauderdale, FL 33304, (305) 463-3867

Fort Myers

- Gary L. Pynckel, DO,
  3940 Metro Parkway, #105, Fort Myers, FL 33916, (813) 278-3377

Holly Hill
- Sam D. Matheny, DO,
  1722 Ridgewood Ave., Holly Hill, FL 32017, (904) 672-2111

Hollywood
- Herbert Pardell, DO,
  210 S. Federal Hwy., #302, Hollywood, FL 33020, (305) 989-5558

Jacksonville
- Allan Spreen, MD,
  5627 Atlantic Blvd., Jacksonville, FL 32207, (904) 645-7585

Jupiter
- Neil Ahner, MD,
  1080 E. Indiantown Rd., Jupiter, FL 33477, (407) 744-0077

Lakeland
- Harold Robinson, MD,
  4406 S. Florida Ave., Suite 27, Lakeland, FL 33803, (813) 646-5088

Lauderdale Lakes
- Daniel Kesden, MD,
  4850 W. Oakland Park Blvd., Suite 257, Lauderdale Lakes, FL 33313, (305) 484-4440

Lauderhill
- Herbert R. Slavin, MD,
  7200 W. Commercial Blvd., Suite 210, Lauderhill, FL 33319, (305) 748-4991

Lighthouse Point
- M. Ginnis, MD,
  2500 N.E. 44th St., Lighthouse Pt., FL 33064, (305) 426-1080

Maitland
- George von Hilsheimer, Ph.D.,
  14 Maitland Plaza, Maitland, FL 32751, (407) 628-0226

Miami
- Martin Dayton, DO,
  18600 Collins Ave., Miami, FL 33160, (305) 931-8484
- Joseph G. Godorov, DO,
  9055 S.W. 87th Ave., Suite 307, Miami, FL 33178, (305) 595-0671
- Renaissance Clinic,
  2972 Coconut Ave., Miami, FL 33133-3726
- Jeffrey Rubin, MD,
  8740 N. Kendall Dr. #210, Miami, FL 33176, (305) 279-1000

North Lauderdale
- Narinder Singh Parhar, MD,
  1333 So. State Road 7, North Lauderdale, FL 33068, (305) 978-6604

North Miami Beach
- Martin Dayton, DO,
  18600 Collins Ave., N. Miami Beach, FL 33160, (305) 931-8484

Ocala
- Sheldon Katanick, DO,
  3405 S.W. College Rd., Ocala, FL 32674, (904) 237-4133

Orlando
- Way, DO,
  500 N. Mills Rd., Orlando, FL 32803, (407) 843-2342

Pensacola
- Ward Dean, MD,
  P.O. Box 11097, Pensacola, FL 32524, (904) 435-5917

Pompano Beach
- Dan C. Roehm, MD,
  3400 Park Central Blvd. N., Suite 3450, Pompano Beach, FL 33064, (305) 977-3700
- Moke W. Williams, MD,
  50 N.E. 26th Ave. #302, Pompano Beach, FL 33062, (305) 782-8855

Port Canaveral
- James M. Parsons, MD,
  Sunstate Preventative, Medicine Institute, Port Canaveral, FL, (407) 784-2102

St. Augustine
- Charles Turner, MD,
  3681 Highway A1A South, St. Augustine, FL 32084, (904) 471-9104

St. Petersburg
- Ray Wunderlich Jr., MD,
  666-6th Street South, St. Petersburg, FL 33408, (813) 822-3612

Stuart
- Richard Plagenhoef, MD,
  3313 S.E. Federal Hwy., Stuart, FL 34997, (407) 288-1000

Tampa
- Eugene H. Lee, MD,
  1804 W. Kennedy Blvd. #A, Tampa, FL 33606, (813) 251-3089

Wauchula
- Alfred S. Massam, MD,
  P.O. Box 1328, 528 West Main St., Wauchula, FL 33873, (813) 773-6668

Winter Park
- Larry T. Martin, DC,
  6906 Aloma Ave, Winter Park, FL 32792, (407) 657-1600
- James M. Parsons, MD,
  Sunstate Preventative, Medicine Institute, Winter Park, FL, (407) 628-3399
- Roger J. Rogers, MD,
  1865 N. Semoran Blvd. #204, Winter Park, FL 32792, (407) 679-2811

GEORGIA

Albany
- O. Jack Woodard, MD,
  1304 Whispering Pines Rd., Albany, GA 31707, (912) 436-9535

Atlanta
- David Epstein, DO,
  427 Moreland Ave., #100, Atlanta, GA 30307, (404) 525-7333
- Milton Fried, MD,
  4426 Tilly Mill Road, Atlanta, GA 30360, (404) 451-4857

- Dr. Bernard Mlaver, M.D.,
  4480 N. Shallow Ford Rd., Atlanta, GA 30338, (404) 395-1600

Camilla
- Oliver L. Gunter, MD,
  24 N. Ellis Street, Camilla, GA 31730, (912) 336-7343

Hazelhurst
- David Turfler, MD,
  111 Cross St., Hazelhurst, GA 31539, (912) 375-3095

Marietta
- Ralph Lee, MD,
  110 Lewis Dr. #B, Marietta, GA 30060, (404) 423-0064
- Norcross, Dr. S. Edelson,
  6920 Jimmy Carter Blvd., Norcross, GA 30071, (404) 729-8359
- Terrill J. Schneider, MD,
  205 Dental Drive, Ste. 3, Warner Robins, GA 31088, (912) 929-1027

HAWAII
Kealakekua
- Clifton Arrington, MD,
  P.O. Box 649, Kealakekua, HI 96750, (808) 322-9400

IDAHO
Coeur d'Alene
- K. Peter McCallum, MD,
  2615 No. 4th St., #609, Coeur d'Alene, ID 83814
- Charles T. McGee, MD,
  1717 Lincolnway, Ste. 108, Coeur d'Alene, ID 83814, (208) 664-1478

Nampa
- John O. Boxall, MD,
  824 - 17th Ave. South, Nampa, ID 83651, (208) 466-3518

Potlatch
- Joan Pierce, DC,
  Potlatch Health Center, 225 6 St, Potlatch, ID 83855, (208) 875-1313

ILLINOIS
Arlington Heights
- Terrill K. Haws, DO,
  121 So. Wilke Road, Suite 111, Arlington Hgts., IL 60005, (708) 577-9451
- Kingsley Medical Center,
  3401 N. Kennicott Ave., Arlington Hgts., IL 60004, (708) 255-8988

Arlington Heights
- William J. Mauer, DO,
  3401 N. Kennicott Ave., Arlington Hghts., IL 60004, (708) 255-8988

Aurora
- Thomas Hesselink, M.D.,
  888 S. Edgelawn Dr. #1735, Aurora, IL 60506, (708) 844-0011

Belvidere
- M. Paul Dommers, MD,
  554 S. Main St., Belvidere, IL 61008, (815) 544-3112

Chicago
- Klatz, DO,
  2434 N. Greenview, Chicago, IL 60614, (312) 528-1000
- Razvan Rentea, MD,
  3354 N. Paulina, Chicago, IL 60657, (312) 549-0101

Evanston
- Theodore TePas, MD,
  1012 Lake Shore Blvd., Evanston, IL 60202, (708) 328-5826

Geneva
- Richard E. Hrdlicka, MD,
  123 South St., #110, Geneva, IL 60134, (708) 232-1900

Glen Ellyn
- Robert S. Waters, MD,
  739 Roosevelt Road, Glen Ellyn, IL 60137, (708) 790-8100

La Grange
- Joseph Nemecek, MD,
  344 Sherwood Ct., La Grange, IL 60525

Metamora
- Stephen K. Elsasser, DO,
  205 S. Engelwood, Metamora, IL 61548, (309) 367-2321

Moline
- Terry W. Love, DO,
  2610-41st Street, Moline, IL 61252, (309) 764-2900

Oak Park
- Paul J. Dunn, MD,
  715 Lake Street, Oak Park, IL 60301, (312) 383-3800

Ottawa
- Terry W. Love, DO,
  645 W. Main, Ottawa, IL 61350, (815) 434-1977

Rolling Meadows
- Thomas L. Stone, MD,
  1811 Hicks Road, Rolling Meadows, IL 60008, (312) 934-1100

Woodstock
- John R. Tambone, MD,
  102 E. South St., Woodstock, IL 60098, (815) 338-2345

INDIANA

Clarksville
- George Wolverton, MD,
  647 Eastern Blvd., Clarksville, IN 47130, (812) 282-4309

Evansville
- Harold T. Sparks, DO,
  3001 Washington Ave., Evansville, IN 47714, (812) 479-8228

Highland
- Cal Streeter, DO,
  9635 Saric Court, Highland, IN 46322, (219) 924-2410

Indianapolis
- David A. Darbro, MD,
  2124 E. Hanna Ave., Indianapolis, IN 46227, (317) 783-5433

Mooresville
- Norman E. Whitney, DO,
  P.O. Box 173, Mooresville, IN 46158, (317) 831-3352

South Bend
- David E. Turfler, DO,
  336 W. Navarre St., South Bend, IN 46616, (219) 233-3840

IOWA

Davenport
- David P. Nebbelong, DO,
  622 E. 38th Street, Davenport, IA 52807, (319) 391-0321
- David P. Nebbeling, DO,
  414 N. Mississippi, Davenport, IA 52726, (319) 381-2033

Sioux City
- Horst G. Blume, MD,
  700 Jennings St., Sioux City, IA 51105, (712) 252-4386

KANSAS

Andover
- Stevens B. Acker, MD,
  310 West Central, #D, P.O. Box 483, Andover, KS 67002, (316) 733-4494

Hays
- Roy N. Neil, MD,
  105 West 13th, Hays, KS 67601, (913) 628-8341

Garden City
- Terry Hunsberger, DO,
  602 N. 3rd - P.O. Box 679, Garden City, KS 67846, (316) 275-7128

Wichita
- Stevens B. Acker, MD,
  P.O. Box 8549, Wichita, KS 67208, (316) 685-3806
- Hugh D. Riordan, MD,
  The Olive Garvey Center, 3100 North Hillside, Wichita, KS 67219, (316) 682-9241

KENTUCKY

Bowling Green
- John C. Tapp, MD,
  414 Old Morgantown Rd., Bowling Green, KY 42101, (502) 781-1483

Elizabethtown
- John D. Rhodes III, MD,
  916 Woodland Drive, Elizabethtown, KY 42701, (502) 765-5921

Lexington
- John H. Parks, MD,
  436 West Second Street, Lexington, KY 40508, (606) 254-9001

Louisville
- Kirk Morgan, MD,
  9105 U.S. Hwy. 42, Louisville, KY 40059, (502) 228-0156

Nicholasville
- Walt Stoll, MD,
  6801 Danville Rd., Nicholasville, KY 40356, (606) 233-4273

Somerset
- Stephen S. Kiteck, MD,
  340 Bogle St., Somerset, KY 42501, (606) 678-5137

LOUISIANA

Baton Rouge
- Steve Kuplesky, MD,
  5618 Bayridge, Baton Rouge, LA 70817

Chalmette
- Saroj T. Tampira, MD,
  812 E. Judge Perez, Chalmette, LA 70043, (504) 277-8991

Lafayette
- Barbara Ardoin, MD,
  123 Ridgeway Dr., Lafayette, LA 70505, (318) 981-8204

Mandeville
- Roy M. Montalbano, MD,
  4408 Highway 22, Mandeville, LA 70448, (504) 626-1985

Newellton
- Joseph R. Whitaker, MD,
  P.O. Box 458, Newellton, LA 71357, (318) 467-5131

New Iberia
- Adonis J. Domingue, MD,
  602 N. Lewis St. #600, New Iberia, LA 70560, (318) 365-2196

New Orleans
- James P. Carter,
  1430 Tulane Avenue, New Orleans, LA 70112, (504) 588-5136

St. Martinsville
- Sidney Dupois, Ph.D.,
  P.O. Box 125, St. Martinsville, LA 70582

MAINE

Brunswick
- Conrad R. Wurtz, Ph.D.,
  18 Center St., Brunswick, ME 04011, (207) 782-1035 or, (207) 729-9916

Van Buren
- Joseph Cyr, MD,
  62 Main Street, Van Buren, ME 04785, (207) 868-5273

MARYLAND

Chevy Chase
- Wyrth Post Baker, MD,
  4701 Willard Avenue, Chevy Chase, MD 20815, (301) 656-8940

Laurel
- Paul V. Beals, MD,
  9101 Cherry Lane Park, Suite 205, Laurel, MD 20708, (301) 490-9911

Randallstown
- Arnold Brenner, MD,
  8622 Liberty Plaza Mall, Randallstown, MD 21133, (410) 922-1133

MASSACHUSETTS

Barnstable
- Michael Janson, MD,
  275 Mill Way, P.O. Box 732, Barnstable, MA 02630, (508) 362-4343

Cambridge
- Michael Janson, MD,
  2557 Massachusetts Ave., Cambridge, MA 02140, (617) 661-6225
- A. William Menzin, MD,
  PC, 56 Alpine Street, Cambridge, MA 02138, (617) 497-0944

Hanover
- Richard Cohen, MD,
  51 Mill St., #1, Hanover, MA 02339, (617) 829-9281

Lenox
- Neil S. Orenstein, PhD,
  77 Church St., Lenox, MA 01240, (413) 637-3466

Newton
- Carol Englender, MD,
  1126 Beacon St., Newton, MA 02161, (617) 965-7770
- Jeanne Hubbuch, MD,
  1126 Beacon St., Newton, MA 02161, (617) 965-7770
- Peggy Roberts, MD,
  1126 Beacon St., Newton, MA 02161, (617) 965-7770

West Boylston
- N. Thomas La Cava, MD,
  360 W. Boylston St., #107, West Boylston, MA 01583, (504) 854-1380

MICHIGAN

Atlanta
- Leo Modzinski, DO, MD,
  100 W. State St., Atlanta, MI 49709, (517) 785-4254

Bay City
- Doyle B. Hill, DO,
  2520 N. Euclid Ave., Bay City, MI 48706, (517) 686-5200
- David Songer, MD,
  4354 E. Wilder Rd., Bay City, MI 48706, (517) 686-1911

Detroit
- John R. Verbovsky, DO,
  19300 Van Dyke, Detroit, MI 48234, (313) 366-2050

Farmington Hills
- Barbara A. Kelly, DC,
  23280 Farmington Rd, Farmington, MI 48336, (313) 474-4484
- Miller, DC,
  31300 Rexwood, Farmington Hills, MI 48016, (313) 932-0200
- Paul A. Parente, DO,
  30275 Thirteen Mile Rd., Farmington Hills, MI 48018, (313) 626-9690
- Albert J. Scarchilli, DO,
  29538 Orchard Lake Rd., Farmington Hills, MI 48018, (313) 626-7544

Flint
- William M. Bernard, DO,
  1044 Gilbert Street, Flint, MI 48532, (313) 733-3140
- Kenneth Ganapini, DO,
  1044 Gilbert St., Flint, MI 48532, (313) 733-3140

Grand Haven
- E. Duane Power, DO,
  P.O. Box 170, Grand Haven, MI 49417, RETIRED

Grand Rapids
- Grant Born, DO,
  2687-44th St. S.E., Grand Rapids, MI 49508, (616) 455-3550

Greenville
- James Nutt, DO,
  420 South Lafayette, Greenville, MI 48838, (616) 754-3679

Lincoln Park
- Kelley, DC,
  3778 Dix Rd., Lincoln Park, MI 48146, (313) 381-8780
- Linares, MD,
  3778 Dix Rd., Lincoln Park, MI 48146, (313) 381-8780

Linden
- Marvin D. Penwell, DO,
  319 S. Bridge Street, Linden, MI 48451, (313) 735-7809

Mt. Pleasant
- John N. Peldyak, DDS,
  611 S. Mission Street, Mt. Pleasant, MI 48858, (517) 773-1250

Pigeon
- David M. Songer, MD,
  7236 Michigan Ave., Pigeon, MI 48755, (517) 453-2020

Pontiac
- Vahagn Agbabian, DO,
  28 No. Saginaw St., Suite 1105, Pontiac, MI 48058-3390, (313) 334-2424

St. Clair Shores
- Richard E. Tapert, DO,
  23550 Harper Avenue, St. Clair Shores, MI 48080, (313) 779-5700

Williamston
- Seldon R. Nelson, DO,
  4386 N. Meridian Rd., Williamston, MI 48895, (517) 349-5346

MINNESOTA

Coon Rapids
- Anne Benassi, DC,
  10666 University Ave., NW, Suite 106, Coon Rapids, MN 55433, (612) 644-1147

Minneapolis
- William Brauer, MD,
  2545 Chicago Avenue, Minneapolis, MN 55404, (612) 871-2611
- Health Recovery Center,
  3255 Hennepin Ave. South, Minneapolis, MN 55408, (612) 827-7800

North Oaks
- Marvin A. Heuer, MD,
  28 Nord Circle, North Oaks, MN 55127, (612) 482-1448

Plymouth
- Jean R. Eckerly, MD,
  10700 Old County Rd. 15, Suite 350, Plymouth, MN 55441, (612) 593-9458

St. Louis Park
- Johnson, DO,
  4820 Excelsior Blvd., #119, St. Louis Park, MN 55416, (612) 920-2942

St. Paul
- Candice Matthiae, DC,
  2301 Como Ave., #202, St. Paul, MN 55108, (612) 644-1147
- Randy Miland, DC,
  7060 Valley Creek Rd., Suite 121, St. Paul, MN 55125, (612) 735-8653

MISSISSIPPI

Clinton
- Walter Evans, Ph.D.,
  102 Midway Dr., Clinton, MS 39056, (601) 924-5605

Coldwater
- Pravindhandra Patel, MD,
  P.O. Drawer DD, Coldwater, MS 38618, (601) 622-7011

Columbus
- James H. Sams, MD,
  P.O. Box 2383, Columbus, MS 39704, (601) 327-8701

Corinth
- Dr. Arnold Smith,
  Magnolia Radiation-Oncology Ctr., 701 Acorn Drive, Corinth, MS 38834-9111,
  (601) 286-4252

Gautier
- David Penton, Ph.D.,
  4113 VanCleave Rd. #2, Gautier, MS 39553, (601) 497-6000

Ocean Springs
- James H. Waddell, MD,
  1520 Government Street, Ocean Springs, MS 39564, (601) 875-5505

Shelby
- Robert Hollingsworth, MD,
  Drawer 87, 901 Forrest St., Shelby, MS 38774, (601) 398-5106

MISSOURI

Clayton
- Walker, Jr., MD,
  138 N. Meramec Ave., Clayton, MO 63105, (314) 721-7227

Festus
- John T. Schwent, DO,
  1400 Truman Blvd., Festus, MO 63028, (314) 937-8688

Florissant
- Tipu Sultan, MD,
  11585 W. Florissant, Florissant, MO 63033, (314) 921-7100
- Garry Vickar, MD,
  1245 Graham Road, Florissant, MO 63031, (314) 837-4900

Independence
- Lawrence E. Dorman, DO,
  9120 E. 35th Street, Independence, MO 64052, (816) 358-2712
- James E. Swann, DO,
  2116 Sterling, Independence, MO 64052, (816) 833-3366

Kansas City
- Edward W. McDonagh, DO,
  McDonagh Medical Center, 2800-A Kendallwood Pkwy., Kansas City, MO 64119,
  (816) 453-5940
- James Rowland, DO,
  8133 Wornall Rd., Kansas City, MO 64114, (816) 361-4077
- Charles Rudolph, DO, Ph.D.,
  2800-A Kendallwood Pkwy., Kansas City, MO 64119, (816) 453-5940

St. Louis
- Rude Suwannasri, MD,
  3009 N. Ballas Rd. #365, St. Louis, MO 63105, (314) 993-3680
- Harvey Walker, Jr., MD, Ph.D.,
  138 N. Meramec Ave., St. Louis, MO 63105, (314) 721-7227

Salem
- Bob R. Carnett, DO,
  P.O. Box 40, Rolla Rd. at McArthur St., Salem, MO 65560, (314) 729-6225

Springfield
- William C. Sunderwirth, DO,
  2828 N. National, Springfield, MO 65803, (417) 869-6260
- G. Fred Warren, DO,
  604 South Pickwick, Springfield, MO 65802, (417) 864-5986

Sullivan
* Ronald H. Scott, DO,
  131 Meredith Lane, Sullivan, MO 63080, (314) 468-4932

MONTANA

Eureka
* Peter R. Rothschild, MD,
  P.O. Box 1290, Eureka, MT 59917

Whitefish
* David V. Kauffman, MD,
  P.O. Box 1837, Whitefish, MT 59937, (406) 862-3961, (Retired)

NEBRASKA

Omaha
* Eugene Oliveto, MD,
  8031 W. Center Road #208, Omaha, NE 68124, (404) 392-0233

NEVADA

Henderson
* Craig Roles, DC, DABCI,
  2720 Green Valley Pkwy., Henderson, NV 89014, (702) 451-0480

Incline Village
* W. Douglas Brodie, MD,
  P.O. Drawer BL, 848 Tanager, Incline Village, NV 89450, (702) 832-7001

Las Vegas
* Richard Baker, MD,
  2200 Rancho Dr., Las Vegas, NV 89102
* Ji-Zhou (Joseph) Kang, MD,
  5613 S. Eastern, Las Vegas, NV 89119, (702) 798-2992
* Robert D. Milne, MD,
  501 S. Rancho, Ste. 446, Las Vegas, NV 89106, (702) 385-1999
* Dan F. Royal, DO,
  3720 Howard Hughes Pk., Suite 270, Las Vegas, NV 89109, (702) 385-7771
* Robert Vance, DO,
  801 S. Rancho Drive, Suite F2, Las Vegas, NV 89106, (702) 385-7771

Reno
* Eric Olkkola, DC,
  2999 S. Virginia St., Reno, NV 89502, (702) 827-5995
* Graham Simpson, MD,
  900 Ryland, Reno, NV 89502, (702) 688-5868
* Donald E. Soli, MD,
  708 North Center St., Reno, NV 89501, (702) 786-7101

NEW HAMPSHIRE

Keene

- Robert Mullaly, Ph.D.,
  Box 404, Keene, NH 03431, (603) 357-4555

NEW JERSEY

Bloomfield

- Majid Ali, MD,
  320 Belleville Ave., Bloomfield, NJ 07003, (201) 743-1151

Boonton Township

- Mary Cody, Ph.D.,
  Box 355A, Meadowbrook Rd., Boonton Township, NJ 07005, (201) 335-9841

Cherry Hill

- Allan Magaziner, DO,
  1907 Greentree Rd., Cherry Hill, NJ 08003, (609) 424-8222

Denville

- Majid Ali, MD,
  95 E. Main St., Denville, NJ 07834, (201) 586-4111
- Walter Burnstein, DO,
  3 Whitman Drive, Denville, NJ 07876, (201) 584-4947

Dunellen

- Edwin Heleniak, MD,
  811 Madison Ave., Dunellen, NJ 08812, (201) 752-2216

Edison

- C.Y. Lee, MD,
  952 Amboy Avenue, Edison, NJ 08837, (201) 738-9220
- Ralph Lev, MD, MS,
  952 Amboy Avenue, Edison, NJ 08837, (201) 738-9220
- Richard B. Menashe, DO,
  15 South Main St., Edison, NJ 08837, (201) 906-8866

Howell

- Steven Streit, MD,
  4710 Hwy. 9, Howell, NJ 07731, (908) 367-5330

Madison

- Michael Westreich DDS, PA,
  18 Madison Avenue, Madison, NJ 07940, (201) 822-0330

Montclair

- Jack Cohen, MD,
  184 Upper Mountain Ave., Montclair, NJ 07042, (201) 239-6688

Paramus

- Linda Choi, MD,
  12-04 Saddle River Rd., Fair Lawn, NJ 07410, (201) 797-9005

Ridgewood

- Harry Panjwani, MD, Ph.D.,
  141 Dayton St. Box 398, Ridgewood, NJ 07451, (201) 447-2033

Skillman

- Sidney Baker, MD,
  862 Rte. 518, Skillman, NJ 08558
- Eric Braverman, MD,
  100-102 Tamarack Cir., Skillman, NJ 08558, (609) 921-1842
- Dr. William K. Kirby,
  43 Tamarack Cir., Skillman, NJ 08558-9659, (609) 921-1773
- Princeton Brain Bio Center,
  862 Route 518, Skillman, NJ 08558, (609) 924-8607

Summit

- Francesca Skoczylas, MD,
  10 Overlook Road #41, Summit, NJ 07901, (908) 273-9566

West Orange

- Faina Munits, MD,
  51 Pleasant Valley Way, West Orange, NJ 07052, (201) 736-3743

NEW MEXICO

Albuquerque

- Harold Cohen, MD,
  Six Wind Northwest, Albuquerque, NM 87120, (505) 898-7115
- Ralph J. Luciani, DO,
  2301 San Pedro N.E., Suite G, Albuquerque, NM 87110, (505) 888-5995
- Gerald Parker, DO,
  6208 Montgomery Blvd. NE, Suite D, Albuquerque, NM 87109, (505) 884-3506
- David Riley, M.D.,
  11600 Cochiti S.E., Albuquerque, NM 87123
- John T. Taylor, DO,
  6208 Montgomery Blvd. NE, Suite D, Albuquerque, NM 87109, (505) 884-3506

Roswell

- Annette Stoesser, MD,
  112 S. Kentucky, Roswell, NM 88201, (505) 623-2444

Santa Fe

- Shirley Scott, MD,
  P.O. Box 2670, Santa Fe, NM 87504, (505) 986-9960

NEW YORK

Bay Shore

- Joseph Chiaramonte, MD,
  649 Montauk Highway, Bay Shore, NY 11706, (516) 665-2700
- Gerald Goldberg, MD,
  1334 Elayne Ave, Bay Shore, NY 11706, (516) 665-0513

Bethpage

- Frank Lobacz, DO, MD,
  4271 Hempstead Turnpike, Bethpage, NY 11714, (516) 731-7222

Brooklyn
- Frank Nochimson, MD,
  36 - 72nd St., Brooklyn, NY 11209, (718) 630-7195
- Richard Schwimmer, MD,
  2635 Nostrand Ave., Brooklyn, NY 11210, (718) 252-3622
- Harold Weiss, MD,
  8002 19th Ave., Brooklyn, NY 11214, (718) 236-2202
- Pavel Yutsis, MD,
  8120 - 19th Ave., Brooklyn, NY 11214, (718) 234-0500

Fishkill
- Luis F. Villamon, MD,
  97 Main Street, Suite #M, Fishkill, NY 12524, (914) 896-4009

Great Neck
- Jose Yaryura-Tobias, MD,
  935 Northern Blvd., Great Neck, NY 11021, (516) 487-7116

Hillsdale
- Vincent Longobardo, MD,
  Route 22, Hillsdale, NY 12519, (518) 325-5300

Huntington
- Serafina Corsello, MD,
  175 E. Main Street, Huntington, NY 11743, (516) 271-0222

Larchmont
- Charles Biller, MD,
  22 Beach Avenue, Larchmont, NY 10538, (914) 834-2185

Lawrence
- Mitchell Kurk, MD,
  310 Broadway, Lawrence, KY 11559, (516) 239-5540

Messena
- Robert Snider, MD,
  HC 61, Box 43D, Messena, NY 13662, (315) 764-7328

Middletown
- Lionel Alboum, MD,
  2 Executive Blvd., #202, Suffern, NY 10901 , (914) 368-4700

New York
- Joseph Caraccilo, DC,
  242 E. 72nd St., #1W, New York, NY 10021, (212) 570-2700
- Serafina Corsello, MD,
  200 W. 57th St., #1202, New York, NY 10019, (212) 517-2222
- Paul R. Dince, MD,
  15 West 81st Street, New York, NY 10024, (212) 288-6580
- Fryer Research Center,
  30 E. 40th St., #608, New York, NY 10016, (212) 808-4940
- Fusco, RN,
  333 E. 43, Suite 114, New York, NY 10017, (212) 983-6383
- Ronald Hoffman, MD,
  40 E. 30th Street, New York, NY 10016, (212) 779-1744

- Warren M. Levin, MD,
  444 Park Ave. So./30th St., New York, NY 10016, (212) 696-1900
- Meduri, Ph.D.,
  239 East 49th St., New York, NY 10017, (212) 752-7111
- Richard Ribner, MD,
  25 Central Park West, New York, NY 10023, (212) 246-7010
- Stanley H. Title, MD,
  171 West 57th Street, New York, NY 10019, (212) 581-9532
- Judith Volpe, MD,
  310 W. 72nd St., #1G, Mew York, NY 10024, (212) 580-3333

Niagara Falls
- Paul Cutler, MD,
  652 Elmwood Ave., Niagara Falls, NY 14301, (716) 284-5140

Old Bethpage
- Terence Dulin, DC,
  735 Old Bethpage Rd., Old Bethpage, NY 11804, (516) 293-4276

Orangeburg
- Neil L. Block, MD,
  14 Prell Plaza, Orangeburg, NY 10962, (914) 359-3300

Plattsburgh
- Driss Hassam, MD,
  50 Court Street, Plattsburgh, NY 12901, (518) 561-2023

Rhinebeck
- Kenneth A. Bock, MD,
  108 Montgomery St., Rhinebeck, NY 12572, (914) 876-7082

Roslyn
- Frederic Vagnini, MD,
  55 Bryant Avenue, Roslyn, NY 11576, (516) 484-6050

Utica
- Tom Bechard, MD,
  4 Hobart St., Utica, NY 13501, (315) 724-8539

Westbury
- Savely Yurkovsky, MD,
  309 Madison St., Westbury, NY 11590, (516) 333-2929

NORTH CAROLINA

Hendersonville
- E. Randall Horton, Jr., DO,
  513 Starmount Lane, Hendersonville, NC 28739

Leicester
- John L. Laird, MD,
  Rt. 1 - Box 7, Leicester, NC 28748, (704) 683-3101

Monroe
- Dennis Reno, DC,
  2204 Commerce Dr., Monroe, NC 28110, (704) 283-7444

NORTH DAKOTA

Grand Forks
- Richard H. Leigh, MD,
  2314 Library Circle, Grand Forks, ND 58201
- Louis Silverman, MD,
  2524 Olson Dr., Grand Forks, ND 58201

Minot
- Brian E. Briggs, MD,
  718 - 6th Street S.W., Minot, ND 58701, (701) 838-6011

OHIO

Akron
- Josephine Aronica, MD,
  1867 W. Market St., Akron, OH 44313, (216) 867-7361

Bluffton
- L. Terry Chappell, MD,
  122 Thurman St., Bluffton, OH 45817, (419) 358-4627

Canton
- Jack E. Slingluff, DO,
  5850 Fulton Rd. N.W., Canton, OH 44718, (216) 494-8641

Centerville
- Heather Morgan, MD,
  138 S. Main St., Centerville, OH 45459, (513) 439-1797

Cincinnati
- Kaushal K. Bhardwaj, MD,
  8325 Colerain Ave., Cincinnati, OH 45239, (513) 741-7467

Cleveland
- John M. Baron, DO,
  4807 Rockside Road, Suite 100, Cleveland, OH 44131, (216) 642-0082
- James P. Frackelton, MD,
  24700 Center Ridge Rd., Cleveland, OH 44145, (216) 835-0104
- Derrick Lonsdale, MD,
  24700 Center Ridge Rd., Cleveland, OH 44145, (216) 835-0104
- Douglas Weeks, MD,
  24700 Center Ridge Rd., Cleveland, OH 44145, (216) 835-0104

Columbus
- Robert R. Hershner, DO,
  1571 E. Livingston Ave., Columbus, OH 43255, (614) 253-8733
- Leonard Kaplan, MD,
  1966 Morse Road, Columbus, OH 43229, (614) 431-9393
- William C. Schmelzer, MD,
  28 W. Henderson Rd., Columbus, OH 43214
- Harold J. Wilson, MD,
  Wilson Medical Center, 4011 Riverview Dr., Columbus, OH 43221, (614) 261-0151

Dayton
- David D. Goldberg, MD,
  100 Forest Park Dr., Dayton, OH 45405, (513) 277-1722

Hubbard
- James Dambrogio, DO,
  212 N. Main Street, Hubbard, OH 44425, (216) 534-9737

Paulding
- Don K. Snyder, MD,
  Route 2 - Box 1271, Paulding, OH 45879, (419) 399-2045

Westlake
- Francis McCafferty, MD,
  31314 Center Ridge Rd., Westlake, OH 44145-5032, (216) 835-3892

Youngstown
- Glenn Kluge, MD,
  1561 Lansdowne Blvd., Youngstown, OH 44505, (216) 743-7787
- James Ventresco Jr., DO,
  3848 Tippecanoe Rd., Youngstown, OH 44511, (216) 792-2349

OKLAHOMA

Choctaw
- William Philpott, MD,
  17171 S.E. 29th St., Choctaw, OK 73020, (405) 390-3009

Edmond
- Vicki J. Conrad, MD,
  1616 S. Boulevard, Edmond, OK 73013, (405) 341-5691

Henryetta
- Brent Wade Davis, DO,
  P.O. Box 207, Henryetta, OK 74437, (918) 299-5038

Jenks
- Leon Anderson, DO,
  121 Second Street, Jenks, OK 74037, (918) 299-5039

Norman
- Huggland, MD,
  2227 W. Lindsey, #1401, Norman, OK 73069, (405) 329-4457

Oklahoma City
- James W. Hogan, DO,
  937 S.W. 89th, Ste. C, Oklahoma City, OK 73139, (405) 631-0524
- Charles H. Farr, MD, Ph.D.,
  8524 S. Western, Suite 107, Oklahoma City, OK 73139, (405) 632-8868
- Charles D. Taylor, MD,
  3715 N. Plassen Blvd., Oklahoma City, OK 73118, (405) 525-7751

OREGON

Elkton
- Moser, Ph.D.,
  27402 State Hwy. 38, Elkton, OR 97436, (503) 584-2325

Eugene
- John Gambee, MD,
  66 Club Road, Ste. 140, Eugene, OR 97401, (503) 686-2536

Grants Pass
- James Fitzsimmons, Jr., MD,
  591 Hidden Valley Rd., Grants Pass, OR 97527, (503) 474-2166

PENNSYLVANIA

Allentown
- Robert H. Schmidt, DO,
  1227 Liberty Plaza Bldg., Suite 303, Allentown, PA 18102, (215) 437-1959

Bala Cynwyd
- Howard Posner, MD,
  111 Bala Avenue, Bala Cynwyd, PA 19004, (215) 667-2927

Bangor
- Francis J. Cinelli, DO,
  153 N. 11th Street, Bangor, PA 18013, (215) 588-4502

Boyerstown
- W. William Shay, DO,
  407 E. Philadelphia Ave., Boyerstown, PA 19512, (215) 367-5505

Elizabethtown
- Dennis L. Gilbert, DO,
  50 North Market Street, Elizabethtown, PA 17022, (717) 367-1345

Greensburg
- Ralph A. Miranda, MD,
  R.D. #12 - Box 108, Greensburg, PA 15601, (412) 838-7632

Hazleton
Arthur L. Koch, DO,
  57 West Juniper St., Hazleton, PA 18201, (717) 455-4747

Indiana
- Chandrika P. Sinha, MD,
  1177 South Sixth Street, Indiana, PA 15701, (412) 349-1414

Mertztown
- Conrad G. Maulfair Jr., DO,
  Box 71 - Main Street, Mertztown, PA 19539, (215) 682-2104

Mt. Pleasant
- Mamduh El-Attrache, MD,
  20 E. Main Street, Mt. Pleasant, PA 15666, (412) 547-3576

North Versailles
- Mamduh El-Attrache, MD,
  215 Crooked Run Road, North Versailles, PA 15137, (412) 673-3900

New Enterprise
- Ella McElwee, MD,
  RD 1, Box 419 A, New Enterprise, PA 16664, (814) 766-3643

North Wales
- Carrie Cossaboon, Ph.D.,
  342 Meadowbrook Rd., North Wales, PA 19454, (215) 699-4600

Philadelphia
- Frederick Burton, MD,
  69 W. Schoolhouse Lane, Philadelphia, PA 19144, (215) 844-4660
- Leander T. Ellis, MD,
  2746 Belmont Avenue, Philadelphia, PA 19131, (215) 477-6444
- P. Jayalakshmi, MD,
  6366 Sherwood Road, Philadelphia, PA 19151, (215) 473-4226
- K.R. Sampathachar, MD,
  6366 Sherwood Road, Philadelphia, PA 19151, (215) 473-4226
- Lance Wright, MD,
  3901 Market Street, Philadelphia, PA 19104, (215) 387-1200

Quakertown
- Harold Buttram, MD,
  RD. #3 - Clymer Road, Quakertown, PA 18951, (215) 536-1890

SOUTH CAROLINA

Columbia
- Theodore C. Rozema, MD,
  2228 Airport Road, Columbia, SC 29205, (803) 796-1702

Landrum
- Theodore C. Rozema, MD,
  1000 E. Rutherford Rd., Landrum, SC 29356, (803) 457-4141, (800) 922-5821 (SC),
  (800) 922-8350 (NAT)

TENNESSEE

Jackson
- Dr. S. Marshall Fram,
  135 Wheatridge Dr., Jackson, TN 38305, (901) 664-0881

Morristown
- Donald Thompson, MD,
  P.O. Box 2088, Morristown, TN 37816, (615) 581-6367

TEXAS

Abilene
- William Irby Fox, MD,
  1227 N. Mockingbird Ln., Abilene, TX 79603, (915) 672-7863

Alamo
- Herbert Carr, DO,
  P.O. Box 1179, Alamo, TX 78516, (512) 787-6668

Amarillo
- Gerald Parker, DO,
  4714 S. Western, Amarillo, TX 79109, (806) 355-8263
- John T. Taylor, DO,
  4714 S. Western, Amarillo, TX 79109, (806) 355-8263

Austin
- Vladimir Rizov, MD,
  Alternative Center, 8235 Shoal Creek , Austin, TX 78758, (512) 451-8149

Brownsville
- Frank Morales, Sr., MD,
  125 Candlewick Court, Brownsville, TX 78521, (512) 546-5752

Dallas
- Brij Myer, MD,
  4222 Trinity Mills Rd., Suite 222, Dallas, TX 75287, (214) 248-2488
- Robert W. Noble, MD,
  6757 Arapaho Road #757, Dallas, TX 75248, (214) 458-9944
- William Rea, MD,
  8345 Walnut Hill Ln. #205, Dallas, TX 75231, (214) 368-4132
- J. Robert Winslow, DO,
  2815 Valley View\Lane, Suite 111, Dallas, TX 75234, (214) 243-7711
- Robert Wilkin, DO,
  200 Webb Royal Plaza, Dallas, TX 75229, (214) 350-2052
- J. Robert Winslow, DO,
  2745 Valwood Pkwy., Dallas, TX 75234, (214) 241-4614

Deer Park
- David Spinks, DO,
  321 W. San Augustine, Deer Park, TX 77536, (713) 476-0780

El Paso
- Edward J. Ettl, MD,
  3500 North Piedras, P.O. Box 31397, El Paso, TX 79931, (915) 566-9361
- Francisco Soto, MD,
  424 Executive Center Blvd., Suite 100, El Paso, TX 79902, (915) 534-0272

Ft. Worth
- Gary H. Campbell, DO,
  7421 Meadowbrook Dr., Ft. Worth, TX 76112, (817) 457-8992

Helotes
- Timothy Werner, DO,
  12910 Bandera Rd., Helotes, TX 78023, (512) 695-3501

Houston
- Robert Battle, MD,
  9910 Long Point, Houston, TX 77055, (713) 932-0552
- Jerome L. Borochoff, MD,
  8830 Long Point, Suite 504, Houston, TX 77055, (713) 461-7517
- Luis E. Guerrero, MD,
  2055 S. Gessner, Suite 150, Houston, TX 77063, (713) 789-0133
- Paul McGuff, MD,
  3838 Hillcroft, Suite 415, Houston, TX 77057, (713) 780-7019

Humble
- John Parks Trowbridge, MD,
  9816 Memorial Blvd., Suite 205, Humble, TX 77338, (713) 540-2329

Kirbyville
- John L. Sessions, DO,
  1609 S. Margaret, Kirbyville, TX 75956, (409) 423-2166

LaPorte
- Ronald Davis, MD,
  10414 W. Main St., LaPorte, TX 77571

Lubbock
- Harlan Wright, DO,
  4903 - 82 St. #50, Lubbock, TX 79424, (806) 792-4811

Midland
- Edison W. McCullough, MD,
  5102 Ashdown Pl, Midland, TX 79705-2801

Pecos
- Richardo Tan, MD,
  423 S. Palm, Pecos, TX 79772, (915) 445-9090

Plano
- Linda Martin-Ernst, DO,
  1524 Independence Pkwy. #C, Plano, TX 75075, (214) 578-1724

Port Arthur
- Robert T. Warhola, DO,
  5885 W. Port Arthur Rd., Port Arthur, TX 77640, (409) 736-2800

San Antonio
- Dr. Jim P. Archer,
  8434 Fredericksburg Rd., San Antonio, TX 78229
- Charles Halff, ND,
  611 Broadway, San Antonio, TX 78215, (512) 226-9003
- Billie Sahley, Ph.D.,
  5282 Medical Dr. #160, San Antonio, TX 78229, (512) 696-1674

Victoria
- George Constant, MD,
  115 Medical Drive #201, Victoria, TX 77904, (512) 576-4182

Wichita Falls
- Thomas R. Humphrey, MD,
  2400 Rushing, Wichita Falls, TX 76308, (817) 766-4329

UTAH
Provo
- Dennis Remington, MD,
  1675 N. 200 West 11E, Provo, UT 84601, (801) 373-8500

VERMONT
Essex Junction
- Charles Anderson, MD,
  175 Pearl Street, Essex Junction, VT 05452, (802) 879-6544

VIRGINIA
Annandale
- Sohini Patel, MD,
  7023 Little River Tnpk., Suite 207, Annandale, VA 22003, (703) 941-3606

Hinton
- Harold Huffman, MD,
  P.O. Box 197, Hinton, VA 22831, (703) 867-5242

McLean
- Henry Palacios, MD,
  1481 Chain Ridge Road, McLean, VA 22101, (703) 356-2244

Midlothian
- Peter C. Gent, DO,
  11900 Hull Street, Midlothian, VA 23112, (804) 744-3551

Norfolk
- Vincent Speckhart, MD,
  902 Graydon Ave, Norfolk, VA 23507, (804) 622-0014

Trout Dale
- Elmer M. Cranton, MD,
  Ripshin Road - Box 44, Trout Dale, VA 24378, (703) 677-3631

WASHINGTON

Bellevue
- Leo Bolles, MD,
  15611 Bel-Red Road, Bellevue, WA 98008, (206) 881-2224
- David Buscher, MD,
  1630-116th Ave., NE, Suite 112, Bellevue, WA 98004, (206) 453-0288
- Maurice L. Stephens, MD,
  15611 Bel-Red Rd., Bellevue, WA 98008, (206) 881-2224

Bellingham
- Robert Kimmel, MD,
  1800 "C" Street, Suite C-8, Bellingham, WA 98225, (206) 734-3250

Edmonds
- Gregory Jantz, Ph.D.,
  Center for Counseling, 611 Main, Edmonds, WA 98020, (206) 771-5166

Freeland
- Donald McCabe, DO,
  1689 E. Main St. #1, Freeland, WA 98249, (206) 321-4424

Kent
- Jonathan Wright, MD,
  24030 - 132nd Ave. S.E., Kent, WA 98042, (206) 631-8920

Kirkland
- Jonathan Collin, MD,
  12911 - 128th St. N.E., Suite F - 100, Kirkland, WA 98034, (206) 820-0547

Port Townsend
- Jonathan Collin, MD,
  911 Tyler Street, Port Townsend, WA 98368, (206) 385-4555

Puyallup
- Robert Bagley, Ph.D.,
  315 39th Ave. SW #11, Puyallup, WA 98373, (206) 848-2242

Seattle
- Donald L. Dudley, MD,
  2825 Eastlake Avenue E., Suite 333, Seattle, WA 98102, (206) 322-0030

- Glen Warner, MD,
  901 Boren #901, Seattle, WA 98104, (206) 292-2277

Spokane
- Burton B. Hart, DO,
  20 South Pines, Spokane, WA 99206, (206) 927-9922

Vancouver
- Richard P. Huemer, MD,
  406 S.E. 131st Ave., Building C-303, Vancouver, WA 98684, (206) 253-4445

Yakima
- Murray L. Black, DO,
  609 S. 48th Ave., Yakima, WA 98908, (509) 966-1780
- Richard Wilkenson, MD,
  302 S. 12th Ave, Yakima, WA 98902, (509) 453-5506

WEST VIRGINIA
Beckley
- Prudencio Corro, MD,
  Route 4 - Box 630, Beckley, WV 25801, (304) 252-0775

Charleston
- Steve M. Zekan, MD,
  1208 Kanawha Blvd. E., Charleston, WV 25301, (304) 343-7559

Iaeger
- Ebb K. Whitley, Jr., MD,
  Route 52 - Box 540, Iaeger, WV 24844, (304) 938-5357

WISCONSIN
Green Bay
- Eleazar M. Kadile, MD,
  1538 Bellevue St., Green Bay, WI 54311, (414) 468-9442

Lake Geneva
- Rathna Alwa, MD,
  717 Geneva Street, Lake Geneva, WI 53147, (414) 248-1430

Milwaukee
- William J. Faber, DO,
  6529 W. Fond du Lac Ave., Milwaukee, WI 53218, (414) 464-7680
- Allen Robertson, Jr. D.O.,
  10520 w. Blue Mound Rd. #202, Milwaukee, WI 53226, (414) 259-1350

Necedah
- Philip F. Mussari, MD,
  P.O. Box 409, 235 Main Street, Necedah, WI 54646, (608) 565-7401

Wisconsin Dells
- Robert S. Waters, MD,
  Race & Vine Streets, Box 357, Wisconsin Dells, WI 53965, (608) 254-7178

AUSTRALIA

Gosford, N.S.W.
* Heather M. Bassett, MD,
  91 Donnison Street, Gosford, N.S.W. 2250, (043) 24 7388

BELGIUM

Antwerpen
* Hubert Prinsen, MD,
  Lamoriniere Straat 147, 2018 Antwerpen, 32-03-2186392
* Rudy Proesmans, MD,
  Rubenslei 17, 2018 Antwerpen, 32-03-2250313

Ghent
* Michel De Meyer, MD,
  Nekkersberglaan 11, 9000 Ghent, 091-22-33-42

Ninove
* Ingrid De Henau, MD,
  Denderhoutembaan 18, 3400 Ninove, 054-323131

St. Niklaas
* A. De Bruyne, MD,
  Ankerstraat 152B, 2700 St. Niklaas, 32-031-7774150

BRAZIL

Amazonas
* Fernando M. de Souza, MD,
  R. Fortaleza 201, Adrianopolis, Manaus, Amazonas, 092-2367733

Curitiba
* Oslim Malina, MD,
  Rua Casemiro de Abreu 32, Curitiba, PR, Brazil 82.000, (041) 252-4395

Osorio-RS
* Jose Valdai de Souza, MD,
  St. Mal Floriano 1012, s/Iron 1 to 9, Osorio-RS 95520, (051) 663-1269

Pelotas-RS
* Antonio C. Fernandes, MD,
  Rua Santa Tecla 470A, Pelotas, RS 96010, 0532-224699

Porto Alegre
* Moyses Hodara, MD,
  Rua Vigario Jose Inacio, 368, Sala 102, Porto Alegre-RS, (0512) 24-3557
* Carlos J.P. de Sa, MD,
  Marcilio Dias - 1056, Porto Alegre-RS 90060, (512) 33 4832 49 3495

Rio de Janeiro
* Helion Povoa Filho, MD,
  Rua Martins, Ferreira, 80, Botafogo, Rio de Janeiro-R.J. 2271, (021) 2665491
* Jose G. Furtado, MD,
  Rua Jardim Botanico, 295 - Terreo, Rio de Janeior-Brasil, (021) 2864800

São Paulo
- Fernando L. Flaquer, MD,
Rua Prof. Artur Ramos 183, cj33, CEP01454 Sao Paulo, 011-211-2019/813-4945,
Fax: 813-4945

CANADA
Blythe
- Richard W. Street, MD,
Box 100 - Gypsy Lane, Blythe, Ont. N0M 1H0, (519) 523-4433

Errington
- George Barber, MD,
Box 234, Errington, B.C., Canada V0R 1V0, (604) 248-8956

Kalowna
- Alex A. Neil, MD,
205 Rutland Road, Kelowna, B.C., Canada V1X 3B1, (604) 765-4117

Newmarket
- Robert L. Gatis, ND,
Natural Health Direct, 17817 Leslie St., #22C, Newmarket, Ont. L3Y 8C6
- Anke Zimmerman, ND,
Natural Health Direct, 17817 Leslie St., #22C, Newmarket, Ont. L3Y 8C6

Smiths Falls
- Clare Minielly, MD,
33 Williams Street E., Smiths Falls, Ont. K7A 1C3, (613) 283-7703

Vancouver
- Donald W. Stewart, MD,
2184 W. Broadway, #435, Vancouver, B.C., Canada V6K 2E1, (604) 732-1348
- Zigurts Strauts, MD,
3077 Granville St., #201, Vancouver, B.C., Canada V6H 3J9

DENMARK
Aarhus
- Bruce P. Kyle, MD,
Sydtoften 35, 8260 Aarhus, 86-293550

Hulmebaek
- Joergen Rugaard, MD,
23 Kystvej, 3050 Humlebaek

Skodsborg
- Bo Mogelvang, MD,
Strandvejen 134, 2942 Skodsborg, 02-80-79-79

Vejle
- Knut T. Flytlie, MD,
Daemningen 70, 7100 Vejle, 05-822020

Virum
- Claus Hancke, MD,
Hjortholmsvej 2A, DK-2830-Virum, 45 42 85 60 06

- Pierre Eggers-Lura, MD,
  Sondervej 39, 2830 DK Virum, 45 42 85 39 61

DOMINICAN REPUBLIC

Santo Domingo
- Antonio Pannocchia, MD,
  Ave. 27 de Febrero, Suite 201, Santo Domingo 6, 565-3259

EGYPT

Cairo
- Elham G. Behery, MD,
  94 Sarwat St., Orman, Cairo, 011-202-3484517

ENGLAND

High St. Nutley, East Sussex
- Steven Rudd, DC,
  Royal Oak Cottage, High St. Nutley, East Sussex, England, TN22 3NN , 0825 713 457

Pagham, West Sussex
- Phillip Lebon, MD,
  3 The Glade, Pagham, West Sussex P021 4SD, 0243-263624

FRANCE

Paris
- Bruno Crussol, MD,
  4 Rue Des Belles Feuilles, 75016 Paris, (331) 47 55 19 19
- Paul Mussarella, MD,
  96 Rue de Miromesnil, 75008 Paris, (1) 45621938

WEST GERMANY

Bad Fussing
- Karl Heinz Caspers, MD,
  Beethovenstrasse 1, D 8397 Bad Fussing, 08531-21001 or, 08531-21004

Rottach-Egern
- Claus Martin, MD,
  P.O. Box 244, 8183 Rottach-Egern, 8022-6415

Werne
- Jens-Ruediger Collatz, MD,
  Fuerstenhofklinik, Fuerstenhof 2, D 4712 Werne, 02389-3883

INDONESIA

Bandung
- Benj. Widjajakusuma, MD,
  Pasirkaliki 115, Bandung 40172, (022) 615277

Jakarta
- Maimunah Affandi, MD,
  Jalan Gandaria 8, Suite 13, Kebayoran-Baru, Jakarta-Selatan, (021) 716927
- Adjit Singh Gill, MD,
  Jalan Tanah Abang V, Suite 27A, Jakarta, (021) 357359
- Yahya Kisyanto, MD,
  71 Diponegoro, Jakarta, (021) 334636

MEXICO
Chihuahua
- H. Berlanga Reyes, MD,
  Antonio de Montes 2118, Col. San Felipe, Chihuahua, Chih. 31240, (95) 141-3-92-71,
  (95) 141-3-92-75

Guadalajara, Jalisco
- Eleazar A. Carrasco, MD,
  Chapultepec Norte 140-203, Guadalajara, Jalisco 44600, 25-16-55
- F. Navares Merino, MD,
  Lopez Mateos Nte. 646, S.H., Guadalajara, Jal. 44680, (36) 16-88-70

Juarez, Chih.
- H. Berlanga Reyes, MD,
  Insurgentes 2516, Cd. Juarez, Chih. 32330, 13-80-23

Matamoros, Tamp.
- Frank Morales, Sr., MD,
  1 a y Nordos, Cal. Jardin, H. Matamoros, Tamp., 3-31-07

Tijuana
- Francisco Rique, MD,
  Azucenas 15, Frac. del Prado, Tijuana, B.C., 011 52 66 813 171
- Rodrigo Rodriguez, MD,
  Azucenas 15, Frac. del Prado, Tijuana, B.C., (706) 681-3171
- Roberto Tapia, MD,
  Azucenas 15, Frac. del Prado, Tijuana, B.C., (706) 681-3171

Torreon, Coahuila
- Carlos Lopez Moreno, MD,
  Tulipanes 475, Col. Torreon, Jardin, Torreon, Coahuila 27200, 011-52-17-138140

NETHERLANDS
Bilthoven
- C.J.M. Broekhuyse, MD,
  Hobbemalaan 11, 3723 EP Bilthoven, 030-250774

Haarlem
- A.M. Jessurun, MD,
  Kenaupark 22, 2011 MT Haarlem, 31-023-328833
- Eduard Schweden, MD, Kenaupark 22, 2011 MT Haarlem, 31-023-328833

Haarzuilens
- C.J.M. Broekhuyse, MD,
  Joostenlaan 1, 3455 SP Haarzuilens, 31-03407-3714

Leende
- Peter van der Schaar, MD,
  Renheide 2, Leende 5595XJ, 31-4959-2232
- Marc Verheyen, MD,
  Renheide 2, Leende 5595XJ, 31-4959-2232

Maastricht
- Rob van Zandvoort, MD,
  Burg. Cortenstraat 26, 6226 GV Maastricht, 31-043-623474

Rotterdam
- Dirk van Lith, MD,
  Zoutmanstraat 4, 3012 EV Rotterdam, 01131 10 4126362/4147633
- Robert T.H.K. Trossel, MD,
  Preventive Medical Center, Joost Banckertsplaats 24-29, 3012 HB Rotterdam, 31 (o) 110 4147633, 31 (o) 10 4147990 FAX Utrecht
- P.J.C. Riethoven, MD,
  Ramstraat 27-A, 3581 HD Utrecht, 030-518951

Velp
- J.H. Leenders, MD,
  344 Arnhemsestraatweg, Velp 6881 NK, 31-085-642742

NETHERLANDS - ANTILLES

St. Maarten
- Danielle Abadjieff, MD,
  9 Almond Grove, Colebay, St. Maarten, 011-5995-442249
- Dirk van Lith, MD,
  P.O. Box 3030, Simpson Bay Corner 35, St. Maarten, 011-5995-53097
- Robert T.H.K. Trossel, MD,
  P.O. Box 3030, Simpson Bay Corner 35, St. Maarten, 011-5995-53097

NEW ZEALAND

Auckland
- R.H. Bundellu, MD,
  173 Tamaki Rd., Otara, Auckland, 011-64-9-2746701
- Kenneth V. McIver, Phd,
  New Zealand Clinic of, Biological Medicine, Dr. Acu, Dip. Hom., 51A Sunset Rd., Ste. A, Glenfield, Auckland 10, New Zealand, (09) 441 0922, (09) 443 0922 (Fax)

Christchurch
- Robert Blackmore, MD,
  196 Hills Road, Christchurch 1, (03) 853-015

Hamilton
- William J. Reeder, MD,
  P.O. Box 4187, Hamilton, (071) 78425

Masterton
- T.J. Baily Gibson, MD,
  P.O. Box 274, Masterton, (059) 81-250

Napier
- Tony Edwards,
  30 Munroe St., Napier, (070) 354-696

New Lynn
- Raymond Ramirez, MD,
  3075 Great North Rd., New Lynn, Auckland, (09) 872-200

Oxford, No. Canterbury
- Ted Walford, MD,
  454 Cameron Road, Tauranga, (075) 86-808

Tauranga
- Michael E. Godfrey, MD,
  Willow House, 14 Willow Street, Tauranga, (075) 782-362

PAKISTAN

Karachi
- M.A. Quraishi, MD, 14B, Hassan Centre, University Rd., Gulshan-e-Iqbal, Karachi,
  219551, 72-69-24 or 72-03-71

PUERTO RICO

Mayaguez
- Leonard Carr, MD, De Diego 10 Oeste, P.O. Box 2045, Mayaguez, PR 00681, (809) 832-3424

Santurze
- Pedro Zayas, MD, P.O. Box 14275, B.O. Librero Station, Santurze, PR,   (809) 727-1105

PHILIPPINES

Manila
- Benjamin P. Aquino, MD,
  Room 406, Singson Bldg., P. Moraga, Binondo, Manila, 47-41-05
- Rosa M. Ami Belli, MD,
  PDC Bldg. Ste. 303-501, 1440 Taft Avenue, Manila, 50-03-23
- Leonides Lerma, MD,
  #301, Pearl Garden, 1700 M. Adriatico Malate, Manila, 57-59-11
- Corazon Macawili-Yu, MD,
  PDC Bldg. Ste. 303-501, 1440 Taft Avenue, Manila, 50-03-23
- Remedios L. Reynoso, MD,
  PDC Bldg. Ste. 303-501, 1440 Taft Avenue, Manila, 50-03-23

SPAIN

Malaga
- Henning Munksnaes, MD,
  Medina Sidonia 192, Urb. Torre Nueva, Mijas Costa/Malaga, 011-34-52-493358

SWITZERLAND

Geneva

- Robert Tissot, MD,
  168 Route de Malagnou, 1224 Geneva, (22) 498875

Basel

- Dr. Sam Baxas,
  Medical Center, Realpstrasse 83, CH - 4054 Basel, (061) 302 90 66

Montreux

- Claude Rossell, MD, Ph.D.,
  Clinique Bon Port, 1820 Montreux, 21-6351-01

Netstal (Glarus)

- Walter Blumer, MD,
  8754 Netstal, (Glarus bei Zurich), 058-61-28-46

TAIWAN

Taipei

- Paul Lin, MD,
  5, Lane 85 Sung Chiang Rd., Taipei, (02) 507-2222 (Taipei), Ext. 1003

WEST INDIES

Jamaica

- H. Marco Brown, MD,
  6 Corna Lane, Montego Bay, Jamaica

APPENDIX B
SUPPLIERS & SERVICES

SUPPLIERS OF PHARMACEUTICALS, VITAMINS AND NUTRIENTS

These listings are provided for information purposes only and are not recommendations by the authors or the publisher. Most suppliers will respond to inquiries about specific products only. Some suppliers offer price lists and order forms upon request. To obtain more information or to order, write or call for ordering information, availability, current prices, and shipping charges. The authors and publisher recommend that readers consult with their physicians before using any products supplied by these companies or any other suppliers.

- Alzheimer's Buyers Club, Box 7006, San Jose 1000, Costa Rica. Organized by Dr. William Summers. Supplies THA and lecithin.
- B. Mougios & Co. O.E., Pittakou 23 T. K., 54645, Thessaloniki, Greece. Supplies most nootropics.
- Baxamed Switzerland Medical Center, Realpstrasse 83, CH-4054 Basel, Switzerland, FAX 061-301-38-72. Supplies smart pharmaceuticals by mail order.
- Big Ben Export Co., Tudor Trading Co., P.O. Box 146, Mill Hill, London NW7 3DL, England. Supplies many smart pharmeceuticals that can be ordered with Visa and Mastercard.
- Cell Tech, 1300 Main St., Klamath Falls, OR. 97601, 503-882-5406. Suppliers of Super Blue-Green™ microalgae products.
- J. Channet, MD, Postfach, CH-891, Rifferswil, Switzerland. Supplies KH-3.
- Discovery Experimental & Development, Mexico, N.A., B & B Freight Forwarding Service, Inc., P.O. Box 7178, Wesley Chapel, FL 33543, 619-661-0010, 619-661-1070, Mexico: 011-5266-304464. Supplies liquid deprenyl which can be ordered COD by phone for 5–7 day UPS delivery.
- Earth Girl's Get Smart Think Drink™, 17370 Skyline Blvd., Woodside, CA 94062; 415-851-9861, 800-783-MIND. Supplies smart drinks products.
- Fountain Research, P.O. Box 250, Lower Lake, CA 95457, 800-659-1915. Supplies liquid deprenyl.
- GH-7 Product Literature, 1920 Monument Blvd. #544, Concord, CA 95420
- Global Medical Information Services, Pharmaceuticals International, 416 West San Ysidro Blvd., #715, San Ysidro, CA 92173. 619-492-8928, 800-365-3698, International 011-52-66-30-0680 for doctor consultation. Offers an extensive catalog of smart products by written request.
- J-M Pharmacal Co. 251-B East Hacienda Ave., Campbell, CA 95008, 408-374-5920, 800-538-4545. Wholesalers of amino acids. Customers can phone for a product and price list.

- Life Services Supplements, Inc., 81 First Avenue, Atlantic Highlands, NJ 07716; 800-542-3230; 908-872-8700; Fax 908-872-8705. Sells Pearson and Shaw products and offers distributorships.

- Longevity Plus Buyer's Club, U Dubu 27, 147 00 Prague 4-Branik, Czechoslovakia. Supplies many smart pharmaceuticals and accepts personal checks. Will send an order form upon request.

- The Mail Order Pharmacy, 3170 North Federal Highway, Suite 104B, Lighthouse Point, FL 33064, 800-822-5388; Fax 800-487-1821. Fills doctor prescriptions by mail order. Patients can consult by phone with the pharmacist who maintains patients' records.

- Masters Marketing Co. Ltd., Masters House, No. 1 Marlborough Hill, Harrow Middx., HA1 1TW, England, Fax 081-427-1994. Supplies a wide range of smart pharmaceuticals and other products. Interested persons must write or Fax specifying information on specific products for a price quotation.

- Mexican pharmacies supply nootropics over the counter without a prescription and are usually less expensive than ordering by mail order.

- Nutritional Engineering, Ltd, Box 1320, Georgetown, Grand Cayman, British West Indies; 800-949-8279; Fax 809-949-7602. Supplies Vitacel products created by Dr. Robert Koch. Customers can order by phone or Fax with a credit card.

- Qwilleran, Box 1210, Birmingham, B10 9QA, England. Supplies most nootropics and some AIDS drugs. Inquiries must specify the products you are interested in.

- Smart Products, 870 Market Street, Suite 1262, San Francisco, CA 94102; Phone: 800-858-6520; Fax 415-981-3334. Supplies smart nutrient products. Orders can be placed by phone with credit card or by mail with personal check. Discounts on orders over $100 and two day delivery is available.

- Sun-Chlorella Ca. Inc., 2641 Manhattan Beach Blvd., Redondo Beach, CA 90278, 213-536-0088. Suppliers of chlorella microalgae products.

- Wholesale Nutrition, Box 3345, Saratoga, CA 95070, 800-325-2664, FAX 408-867-6236. Supplies smart nutrients. Orders can be placed by phone with credit card. Two day delivery is available.

- World Health Services, P.O. Box 20, CH-2822 Courroux, Switzerland. Supplies many European pharmaceuticals that have not been approved by the FDA.

SUPPLIERS ON FDA IMPORT-ALERT LIST

On January 29, 1992, the FDA issued an import alert against six overseas companies. U.S. Customs is instructed to automatically detain all shipments from these companies. The FDA states that these companies were found to be promoting their products in the U.S., or were shipping orders larger than the personal three month supply allowed by the FDA. The import alert confirmed that the FDA would maintain its policy of allowing shipments of small quantities of unapproved drugs for personal use. However, the FDA emphasized that this is a policy and not a law, which means that permitting shipments to pass through U.S. customs is left to the discretion of the FDA's field offices. In short, any shipment of unapproved drugs can be detained arbitrarily.

- Azteca Trio International, S.A. de C.V. in Mexico.

- Interlab, BC, Box 5890, London, WCIN 3XX, England. & Box 587, Newport Pagnell, Bucks MK16 8AA, England.

- InHome Health, Box 3112, CH 2800 Dalemont, Switzerland.
- Interpharm, Inc in the Bahamas.
- International Products in Germany.
- Northam Medication Service International Pharmacy in the Bahamas.

SERVICES

The following listing of services is provided for information purposes only and is not recommended by the authors or publisher. Readers should contact service providers directly for program literature and then consult their physicians before enrolling in any program or using any products.

- Aslan Institute, Inc., Miami, FL; 800-833-9834. Residential program providing traditional Ana Aslan treatment.
- American College of Advancement in Medicine, Box 3427, Laguna Hills, CA 92654. 714-583-7666 or 800-532-3688. Maintains a list of physicans with expertise in life extension and cognative enhancement.
- Earth Girl's Get Smart Think Drinks™, 17370 Skyline Blvd., Woodside, CA 94062; 415-851-9869; 800-783-MIND. Provides a smart bar with smart drinks for events.
- Life Extension Foundation, 2490 Griffin Rd., Ft. Lauderdale, FL 33012; Box 229120, Hollywood, FL 33022; 305-966-4886, 800-841-5433. Members receive monthly newsletter, discounts at The Mail-Order Pharmacy, helpful directories to life extension doctors and innovative medical clinics. Membership is $50.
- Nutrient Café Smart Drinks, Chris Beaumont, Box 170156, San Francisco, CA 94117. 415-267-6178. Provides a smart bar with smart drinks for events. Offers a smart bar recipe book for $2.
- Smart Bars For Hire, Smart Products, 870 Market Street, Suite 1262, San Francisco, CA 94102; 800-858-6520; Fax 415-981-3334. Provides a smart bar and smart drinks for events and recipes for people putting on their own smart bars.
- Dr. William Summers, 624 West Duarte Rd., Suite 101, Arcadia, CA 91007; 818-445-6196; Fax 818-445-4204. Works with families of Alzheimer's patients and affiliated with the Alzheimer's Buyers Club.

INDEX

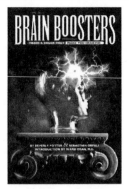

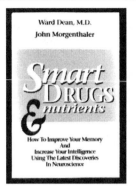

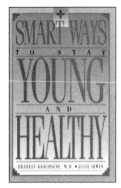

Brain Boosters: Foods & Drugs That Make You Smarter Potter & Orfali. 1993. Fascinating look at foods and drugs that are reported to make the mind work better. For professionals, business people, seniors, people concerned with Alzheimer's and other neurological impairments, as well as students, athletes and party goers who want to improve mental permormance.
Ronin   256pp.
BRABOO $12.95

Smart Nutrients Hoffer & Walker. 1993. Guide to nutrients that can enhance intelligence and reverse senility. Latest nutrition research to strengthen brain power and maintain it throughout a long life. Prevent and correct degenerative brain diseases and improve already strong mental capacities.
Avery   196pp.
SMANUT $9.95

Smart Drugs & Nutrients Dean. 1990. Introductory guide to developments in neuroscience that sparked the smart drug phenomenon. By using nutrients, new compounds, and pharmaceuticals, one may vastly improve memory, concentration, and ability to learn. Volumes 1 & 2 now available.
B&J   188pp.
SMART $12.95
SMART2 $14.95

Neuroendocrine Theory of Aging and Degenerative Disease Dilman and Dean. 1992. Study which suggests that major degenerative diseases arise as a by-product of development and occur in a predictable pattern.
Ctr of Bio-Gerontology 356pp.
NEUTHE $50.00

Biological Aging Measurement Dean. 1990. Clinical approach to health improvement programs by measuring biological age & rates of aging.
Ctr of Bio-Gerontology 426pp.
BAGING $40.00

Smart Ways to Stay Young & Healthy Gascoigne. 1991. Sound advice on how to maintain physical and mental health. Brief chapters, each presenting one simple thing you can do for your well being, youthfulness, and happiness.
Ronin   128pp
SMAWAY $5.95

Mind Food and Smart Pills Pelton. 1989. Sourcebook for vitamins, herbs, and drugs that can increase intelligence, improve memory and prevent brain aging. For students and workers seeking a competitive edge, seniors concerned about maintaining mental powers, and people who have used alcohol or other drugs.
Doubleday   336pp
MFOOD $12.95

Life Extension: A Practical Scientific Apporaach Pearson. 1983. Guide to methods of living longer. Causes of aging, theory and practice of life extension, improving quality of life in sickness and health, nutrients and drugs that prolong life, set up a life extension program.
Warner   896pp
LIFEEXT $14.95

Books by Phone Box 522 Berkeley CA 94701 (800) 858-2665 (510) 548-2124